# Reversing Dry Eye Syndrome

YALE UNIVERSITY PRESS **HEALTH & WELLNESS**

A Yale University Press Health & Wellness Book is an authoritative, accessible source of information on a health-related topic. It may provide guidance to help you lead a healthy life, examine your treatment options for a specific condition or disease, situate a healthcare issue in the context of your life as a whole, or address questions or concerns that linger after visits to your healthcare provider.

Thomas E. Brown, Ph.D., *Attention Deficit Disorder: The Unfocused Mind in Children and Adults*

Ruth H. Grobstein, M.D., Ph.D., *The Breast Cancer Book: What You Need to Know to Make Informed Decisions*

James W. Hicks, M.D., *Fifty Signs of Mental Illness: A Guide to Understanding Mental Health*

Mary Jane Minkin, M.D., and Carol V. Wright, Ph.D., *A Woman's Guide to Menopause and Perimenopause*

Mary Jane Minkin, M.D., and Carol V. Wright, Ph.D., *A Woman's Guide to Sexual Health*

Catherine M. Poole, with DuPont Guerry IV, M.D., *Melanoma: Prevention, Detection, and Treatment,* 2nd ed.

E. Fuller Torrey, M.D., *Surviving Prostate Cancer: What You Need to Know to Make Informed Decisions*

Steven L. Maskin, M.D., with Pamela Thomas, *Reversing Dry Eye Syndrome: Practical Ways to Improve Your Comfort, Vision, and Appearance*

# Reversing Dry Eye Syndrome

## Practical Ways to Improve Your Comfort, Vision, and Appearance

**STEVEN L. MASKIN, M.D.**

WITH PAMELA THOMAS

WITH A FOREWORD BY SCHEFFER C. G. TSENG, M.D., Ph.D.

YALE UNIVERSITY PRESS/NEW HAVEN & LONDON

The information and suggestions contained in this book are not intended to replace the services of your physician or caregiver. Because each person and each medical situation is unique, you should consult your own physician to get answers to your personal questions, to evaluate any symptoms you may have, or to receive suggestions on appropriate medications.

The author has attempted to make this book as accurate and up-to-date as possible, but it may nevertheless contain errors, omissions, or material that is out-of-date at the time you read it. Neither the author nor the publisher has any legal responsibility or liability for errors, omissions, out-of-date material, or the reader's application of the medical information or advice contained in this book.

Published with assistance from the Louis Stern Memorial Fund.



Designed by Mary Valencia.
Set in Stone types by Keystone Typesetting, Inc.
Printed in the United States of America.

ISBN: 978-0-300-12285-5 (pbk.)
978-0-300-11176-7 (cloth)

Library of Congress Control Number: 2006052803
Yale University Press Health & Wellness Series.

A catalogue record for this book is available from the British Library.

The paper in this book meets the guidelines for permanence and durability of the Committee on Production Guidelines for Book Longevity of the Council on Library Resources.

10 9 8 7 6 5 4 3 2 1

*To my mom and dad,*
*Dorothy and Sol Maskin,*
*for their support throughout the years—*
*I love you both more than words can say*

# CONTENTS

# FOREWORD

Why are my eyes irritated, sandy, and itching? Why did my eyes become so uncomfortable all of a sudden after menopause, after wearing contact lenses for many years, or after LASIK surgery? Why do my eyes still burn so after I've seen several eye doctors and had many kinds of eyedrops? These are questions frequently asked by dry eye sufferers.

Dry eye (or dysfunctional tear) syndrome is one of the most common eye diseases, and affects close to 10 percent of the U.S. and European populations. At a mild stage, dry eye presents as an annoying nuisance, but at a moderate stage, it can notably hamper one's ability to function on a daily basis; at a severe stage, it can lead to a permanent loss of vision. The incidence of dry eye is climbing yearly in part because of the introduction of LASIK, a popular eye laser surgery, in the last decade. Despite the fact that dry eye raises an important ocular health issue, until now there has been no lay book devoted solely to unlocking the complexity of the disease and to providing useful guidance for dry eye sufferers.

To address these questions, Dr. Steven Maskin first lays a solid foundation by explaining the importance of tears in maintaining comfort, vision, and appearance. He then details how dry eyes can be caused by factors such as contact lenses, allergy, LASIK surgery, aging, diet, and hormones. In each chapter, he draws the reader's attention by demystifying the conventional wrong belief, then highlighting an exemplary patient drawn from his own clinical practice. While explaining the causative factors of each specific type of dry eye, Dr. Maskin never forgets to extrapolate the scientific essence to the patient's realism. He carefully chooses lay words and plain language after thoughtful distillation of scientific literature. He concludes the book by providing practical guidance for dry eye sufferers so that they may cope with and gain relief from this annoying eye irritation both at home and at work.

Clearly, Dr. Maskin wrote this book with strong passion. It is a passion that I recognized more than fifteen years ago when he received subspecialty clinical fellowship training with us at the Bascom Palmer Eye Institute, Department of Ophthalmology, University of Miami School of Medicine. I wondered then why he took a special interest in dry eye, a disease that at the time was receiving little attention from eye care professionals. He went on to spend another two years in my laboratory studying the basic cell biology of the meibomian glands, which produce essential oily tears in the eye but even today do not receive much attention. As he began his clinical practice in the Tampa area, unlike most of his peers he decided to focus on diseases related to tears and the eye surface instead of more common afflictions such as cataract. I am pleased to see that Dr. Maskin has translated his passion into words by unselfishly sharing his knowledge by means of this book.

Scheffer C. G. Tseng, M.D., Ph.D.

# PREFACE

When I first started looking for a publisher for this book, quite a few people seemed rather dubious. Several editors looked at my initial proposal and inquired, albeit kindly, "What can you possibly have to say about dry eye? Is there really a whole book here?" Fortunately I eventually found an agent, and an editor, who recognized the scope and importance of this topic, and I was able to proceed. Since you are now holding this book in your hands, you can see that, yes, there is "a whole book" about dry eye syndrome. Also, since you are reading this book, you may well suffer from dry eye syndrome yourself, and therefore you know firsthand how painful and frightening it can be.

I have been a practicing ophthalmologist (a medical doctor with a specialty in eye diseases) in Tampa, Florida, for more than fifteen years. Not long after I started practicing, I noticed that more and more patients were coming to see me each year with varying degrees of eye pain. More often than not, this eye pain was the result of a complex disease known as dry eye syndrome. (A recent professional paper suggested that the disease be renamed dysfunctional tear syndrome—which, in fact, more nearly describes its nature. However, since at this time most people recognize the disease as "dry eye syndrome," I will use that label throughout the book.)

Having specialized in ocular surface diseases in my postresidency ophthalmology fellowships, I had learned about the complexities of dry eye syndrome. I already knew from my residency that it was relatively common among patients suffering from Sjögren's syndrome and other serious autoimmune diseases, such as lupus and diabetes. Also, I was well aware that many older people, especially menopausal women, often developed dry eye, now felt to be the result of a hormonal imbalance.

It was evident that many of the causes of dry eye syndrome among my patients paralleled certain advances in medicine and technology. For example, patients who had comfortably worn contact lenses for decades seemed to progressively develop dry eye, even those patients who had changed to the new extended-wear lenses. Or people whose professions (such as accounting or journalism) demanded that they spend several hours each day in front of a computer screen seemed to be complaining of dry eye pain more and more frequently—apparently in direct proportion to the amount of time they spent on their computers. Finally, I was concerned about the number of patients who were experiencing eye pain and serious vision disturbances as a result of LASIK surgery, the relatively new procedure to permanently correct nearsightedness and farsightedness. (Even though the percentage of patients reported to have ongoing problems due to LASIK is quite small, substantial numbers of people were suffering.)

Based on my reading of professional journals, attendance at medical conferences, and talks with colleagues, I could see that I was not alone in my observation that the numbers of people suffering from dry eye syndrome seemed to be growing at an extraordinary rate. Actually, I have had to manage my own issues with dry eye over my 47 years. My mother tells me I first began wearing spectacles when I was 8 years old. When I was 15, while playing basketball my glasses were smashed by an errant shoulder (of a player I was guarding while trying to take away the ball); the metal hinge lacerated my left brow, just missing my eye. My parents switched me to contact lenses, first hard then soft, and I have been wearing contacts ever since.

Sensation in my cornea became mildly diminished after years of contact lenses, and about eight years ago I developed mild to moderate dry eyes. Frequent use of artificial tears began to interfere with my busy daily routine, so I underwent an inferior (lower) punctal occlusion using thermocautery of each eye. I have had very little trouble ever since, only rarely needing to supplement with artificial tears. To avoid problems, I remain cognizant of my environment (steering clear of restaurant fans, for example) and make every effort to avoid other preventable causes of dry eye.

Statistics now show that approximately 9 million Americans suffer from moderate to severe dry eye syndrome, and that number is probably only half the total number of Americans plagued with mild cases of dry eye, who aren't even aware they have the disorder. But make no mistake: this is not only a problem in America. Studies in Denmark and Australia also suggest that close to 10 percent of their populations have at least mild dry eye. What's more, the number is growing.

Suddenly dry eye syndrome is being talked about everywhere. Professional conferences help eye care professionals diagnose and treat various aspects of the disease. Countless studies are being published on an enormous range of topics related to dry eye—from the success of flaxseed supplements in easing dry eye pain, to the reintroduction of a procedure called ocular surface reconstruction with amniotic membrane to treat the damaged conjunctiva that results from severe dry eye. In addition, the first medication purely for the treatment of dry eye, a drop called Restasis, has met with tremendous success.

Despite the clamor today about dry eye, it came to my notice that although several excellent books for ophthalmologists, optometrists, and other eye care professionals were available, no book for the average lay person—the dry eye sufferer!—was on the market. And although a number of websites were accessible on the Internet, I felt it was difficult for a general reader to find the most helpful information.

In my practice I have found that a patient's knowledge about his or her disease or disorder is one of my most useful aids in making a proper diagnosis and prescribing appropriate treatment. The more a patient knows about the physiology of the eye, the causes of the dry eye problem (and any other health problems he or she may have), and the various opportunities for treatment, the more effectively that patient and I can team up to find the best solutions for the problems. This is especially true for dry eye syndrome, which can have many causes and may require a variety of treatments.

With this book, I hope to share my experience treating dry eye in all its types and severity. Although this is not a "medical textbook," it contains a number of scientific descriptions and theories, all of which I have tried to present in a straightforward, easy-to-understand manner useful to the general reader. *Reversing Dry Eye Syndrome* is not encyclopedic (and dry eye can be an *endlessly* complex problem), but I have tried to at least touch on virtually every facet of this disorder, from definition, to causes, to diagnosis and treatment—both medical and home remedies. Remember, though, that this book is not meant to replace your personal eye doctor, but rather to equip you, or anyone suffering with dry eye, with as much up-to-date information as possible so that you too can better work with your ophthalmologist to find complete relief.

Over the years, the following doctors have served as mentors for me, and I am exceedingly grateful to them: Richard Reider, Donald Bode, Wichard Van Heuven, Richard Yee, and Scheffer C. G. Tseng. Dr. Tseng in particular has greatly influenced and encouraged me in my career. It is especially fitting that he has written the foreword to this book, and I thank him for it.

I also thank the members of my office staff who have joined me in caring for our numerous patients, as well as providing secretarial support during the writing of this book: Maria Bautista, Eloise Eggers, Rotonda Green, and Harriet McCranie.

Numerous patients have allowed me to share their stories of painful, dry eyes. Specifically, I thank Claudia Jenkins, Shirley Gilleland, Mary Leah Brainard, Don Polston, Mary Jean Rappelt, Barbara Debrun, Eva Fogarty, and Eric Hinze. Others asked that their names not be used, but I want them to know that I appreciate their generosity and support.

I am grateful for the support and advice of my agent, Ed

Knappman, and of my editor at Yale University Press, Jean Thomson Black, and her assistant, Laura Davulis. Particular thanks go to Pamela Thomas, who persevered while learning about—and then writing about—this very complex disease. Pam, congratulations on a job well done. And my gratitude goes to Alison Schroeer, of Schroeer Scientific Illustration (www.scientificillustration.com), for creating the three explanatory figures in the text.

Finally, of course, I am especially grateful for the understanding and patience of my family during the many months it took to write this book. Very special thanks go to my mom and dad, Dorothy and Sol Maskin; my wife, Angela; and my sons, Benjamin, Jacob, and David, and my daughter, Sarah.

# Reversing Dry Eye Syndrome

CHAPTER

# 1

# What Is Dry Eye Syndrome, and Who Gets It?

Myth

*Dry eye syndrome is not a serious disease.*

Fact

*If dry eye syndrome is not treated properly, it can lead to severe eye problems, including blindness.*

Sandy, aged 48, says her eyes are so red, dry, and irritated that it has become difficult for her to drive, even if she is wearing dark sunglasses. She's been meaning to see her eye doctor, but has put it off. In the meantime she has been relying heavily on over-the-counter eyedrops bought at her local pharmacy. They don't help. In fact her eyes hurt when she puts the drops in, but the bottle said the contents were for dry and irritated eyes, and her eyes certainly fit that description. Maybe after a while, Sandy hopes, pain relief will kick in.

Carl, 42, has been treated with insulin since he was first diagnosed with Type I diabetes at the age of 16. Lately he has noticed a painful, gritty feeling in his eyes. For the last few months, he's been a little lax (well, okay, *very* lax) about keeping his glucose levels down, so he figures that if he just watches his diet more carefully, then the pain in his eyes will disappear as well.

Marie, 28, has been wearing contact lenses since she was 15 years old, but lately they just don't feel right. She takes them out, cleans and wets them, and puts them back in, over and over; but in just a few minutes, the pain bothers her so much that she has to remove her contacts yet again. Marie has been thinking that wearing contacts just isn't worth it. She is nearsighted and doesn't own a pair of conventional glasses (she thinks they would make her look ugly). Lately she has been wondering whether she should see that eye doctor she has heard about who performs LASIK (laser in situ keratomileusis) surgery.

Arthur, 84, suffers from Parkinson's disease. As a direct result of the disease, he doesn't blink with regularity, which would normally lubricate and cleanse his eyes. Crusting frequently builds up around his lashes and lids, and results in constant feelings of grittiness, discomfort, and pain. He has used over-the-counter eyedrops and rinses to try to alleviate the problem, but he is unable to administer the drops on his own and his wife has trouble helping him. Arthur also has trouble physically just getting around, but he attributes his problems solely to the Parkinson's disease and does not realize that dry eye, including a distinct loss of vision, is strongly exacerbating his other issues.

As an ophthalmologist who has treated thousands of patients, I know that millions of people—men and women, young people and old, some suffering from chronic illness and others who are otherwise perfectly healthy—urgently need treatment for dry eye syndrome. Some may not even know it! Sandy, Carl, Marie, and Arthur are typical of many patients I have had. (I will be discussing a number of my patients in this book, but I will not be using their actual names, although their symptoms and problems are real.)

Sandy is using over-the-counter drops that not only are not helping her, but ultimately are increasing her pain. For starters, she needs to stop using the commercial eyedrops. She needs to see an eye doctor as soon as possible to find out why her eyes are hurting so much and to obtain proper treatment. The problem may be that she is allergic to—or, at least sensitive to—the preservatives in the artificial tears.

Carl is correct that he should get his blood-sugar level as close to normal as possible. Diabetes can cause many eye complications, from dry eye syndrome to blindness, as well as other noneye problems such as heart attack and stroke. However, Carl shouldn't assume that improving his blood-sugar level will make his eye problems instantly vanish, nor should he assume that he can handle this problem on his own. He needs to consult with both an endocrinologist for his diabetes and an eye doctor to resolve his dry eye syndrome.

If Marie follows through on her plan to have LASIK surgery to improve her nearsightedness (that is, if she can even find an eye doctor who would be willing to operate on her severely dry eyes), she is at high risk of augmenting the problem she already faces. Maybe Marie can't wear contact lenses any more. Or perhaps she simply needs a different type of contact lens, one that allows for better hydration of her eyes. She also may require minor surgery (usually an in-office procedure) to increase her tear volume and comfort her eyes.

Arthur sees a neurologist regularly to keep his Parkinson's disease under control, yet continues to complain about stumbling and has trouble seeing properly. It hasn't occurred to him, his wife, or even his primary-care physician, that he could benefit by being actively treated for dry eye. All have simply assumed that his problems are Parkinson's related. He should consult with an eye specialist as soon as possible.

## WHAT IS DRY EYE SYNDROME?

If you are reading this book, no doubt you at least suspect that you have chronically dry eyes, or very possibly you have been diagnosed with dry eye syndrome, indicating that your problem has reached a crucial point. My primary goals here are to help you reduce your eye pain and irritation; improve your vision; and possibly even eliminate the redness from your eyes, making you look better. To achieve these ends, I aim to supply you with all the information you'll need in order to deal with your dry eye problem. This includes guiding you toward working effectively with your eye doctor.

Dry eye syndrome, known medically as *keratoconjunctivitis sicca,* is an umbrella term for a condition of severely dry eyes caused by a lack of proper tear production and distribution. (Recently, some experts have recommended that the label "dry eye syndrome" be changed to "dysfunctional tear syndrome." The term "dry eye syndrome" connotes different things to both physicians and to patients, and "dysfunctional tear syndrome" is considered by some experts to be more consistent with the basic issue, which is the diminished quality and quantity of tears. The term "dry eye" suggests that dryness is present in all patients, which is not necessarily the case. Still, for the purposes of this book, I have chosen to call the disorder by its best-known label: dry eye syndrome.)

Basically, dry eye syndrome manifests in one of two ways: aqueous tear deficient dry eyes or evaporative dry eyes. Aqueous tear deficient dry eye develops because the lacrimal (tear) glands, located under the eyelids, do not produce enough tears to keep the surface of the eye sufficiently moist. Evaporative dry eye results from an abnormality in tear composition causing the tears to evaporate too quickly (all of this will be discussed in detail in Chapter 3).

If you have dry eye syndrome, you are well aware that it can be extremely painful. In addition, dry eye syndrome impedes vision by generating blurriness and visual distortion. Glasses don't help because the problem lies with the physical dryness. Contact lenses don't help; in fact, they may make the situation worse because contact lenses need the lubrication of tears to work effectively. Without sufficient tears, contacts often feel like they're painfully glued onto your eyes—as if you are wearing a salty potato chip instead of a contact lens.

Dry eye can severely affect virtually every aspect of your life, from the simplest everyday occurrence to the progress of your career. Experts have found that, with severe dry eye, the decrease in the quality of life is comparable to that among patients with severe angina or a disabling hip fracture. For example, many patients with dry eye syndrome must plan ahead carefully before embarking on the most simple everyday activities, from going to a movie or play, to enjoying dinner in a restaurant, even to riding in a car. They must be sure their eyes are sufficiently lubricated and that they avoid sitting near a heating duct, air-conditioning unit, fan, or any other place where the ambient air is agitated. Not surprisingly, severe dry eye sufferers should avoid smoke-filled rooms and socializing with smokers. They even need to think about the weather as it pertains to their eyes, since wind, rain, and dry or cold conditions affect chronically dry and irritated eyes.

Many patients with dry eye syndrome are dismayed by their deteriorating appearance, for their eyes can often be red and even teary. Often family members, friends, and colleagues begin to notice the sufferer's red, irritated eyes. While most people will be sympathetic, others (one's boss, for example) may mistakenly conclude that the person with the bloodshot eyes must have a serious drug or alcohol problem.

Most seriously, a moderate to severe case of dry eye syndrome can affect the quality of one's work and ultimately the progress of one's career. This is particularly true for anyone who spends several hours each day working on a computer terminal. In this day and age, that includes many, many workers—from lawyers, bankers, accountants, journalists, and writers, to office workers of virtually every stripe. Dry eye can make work that involves the eyes very painful, and, if the dry eye is not dealt with properly, work may become impossible.

## WHAT ARE THE SYMPTOMS?

Everyone has itchy or irritated eyes once in a while, and you shouldn't panic if your eyes occasionally feel a little gritty and inflamed. Conversely, if you develop severe, constant eye pain, call your eye doctor immediately to rule out a neurologic cause such as stroke, a corneal ulcer, a glaucoma attack, or some other serious problem.

Cases of dry eye usually begin with mild symptoms, and the first line of defense for most sufferers is over-the-counter eyedrops or artificial tears. These will treat the symptoms, but don't necessarily alter the progress of the disease. If your eyes are annoyingly scratchy, irritated, and/or inflamed for more than a week or two, have an eye doctor check them.

Listed below are the key symptoms of dry eye syndrome. You may well have dry eye syndrome if you experience only one or two of them; in extreme cases, you may suffer from most or even all of them.

Eye pain, such as achy or sore eyes
Redness of the eyes, inflammation
Scratchy, grainy, gravelly feelings in the eyes
Sense of a "foreign body" in the eyes
Burning or stinging in the eyes
Constant or frequent itching of the eyes
Contact lens discomfort
Nighttime dryness
Difficulty opening your eyes in the morning because they feel glued shut
Frequent blurred or fluctuating vision
Heavy or tired eyes
Excessively watery eyes
Excessive mucus discharge from the eyes
Sensitivity to light

## Eye Pain

Eye pain is probably the most debilitating symptom of dry eye syndrome. Sometimes the pain is so excruciating that you can't open your eyes; you constantly squint for some relief. Eye pain develops because the cornea is extremely sensitive, and when it is not protected by tears, its nerves become exposed. Sometimes the pain is unremitting.

### Redness or Inflammation

Eye redness isn't always caused by dry eye syndrome; it can also result from infections, trauma, lack of sleep, alcohol abuse, or medications. However, many people with dry eye syndrome have at least some degree of eye redness and inflammation, and the redness can be extreme in some patients. Because dry eyes aren't getting lubricated sufficiently with tears, the lids in effect create a "mechanical trauma" with each blink, which results in inflammation of the surface of the eye. Researchers have been investigating this mechanical aspect of dry eye and the resulting inflammation, and have recently recommended new treatments based on their findings, including the first prescription medication specifically to address dry eye symptoms.

### Scratchiness

Many dry eye sufferers experience a sense of scratchiness in their eyes, as if something is abrading the surface of their eyes.

### Foreign Body Sensation

Another common symptom of dry eye is the constant sensation that a foreign body, such as an eyelash or a piece of dirt, is lodged in the eye. The feeling can be simply annoying or excruciatingly painful, but no matter how much you rub or rinse the eye, the sensation remains. Sometimes a piece of mucus has attached itself to the eye, or the cornea may be swollen. Often no actual foreign body exists; instead, the cornea has become more sensitized as a result of the dryness.

### Burning or Stinging

If burning or stinging of the eyes is your problem, you may suffer from evaporative dry eye and require special therapies to obtain relief. At the same time, burning or stinging could mean that you have an allergy that needs to be identified and treated.

### Constant or Frequent Itching

An aggravating sort of itching can be another symptom of dry eye syndrome, especially if you suffer from allergies. This symptom can be exacerbated by rubbing your eyes. The rubbing will not help the itchy feeling go away; besides, the mechanical trauma of rubbing may increase inflammation and thus aggravate your risk for more itching or for developing an eye infection as your fingers transport germs into the normally sterile environment of the eye. Dry eye also allows for increased concentration of allergens to collect on the surface of the eye, resulting in a feeling of itchiness.

### Contact Lens Discomfort

Many people who have worn contact lenses for years develop dry eye, the obvious symptom being that wearing their contacts becomes extremely uncomfortable. This can be true not only with old-fashioned gas-permeable hard lenses, but with soft lenses as well. The symptoms may manifest as irritation or pain.

### Nighttime Dryness

Many patients with dry eye syndrome have serious problems with nighttime dryness of their eyes. The cause may be a problem called nocturnal lagophthalmos, or incomplete eye closure during sleep.

### Difficulty Opening Your Eyes in the Morning

Difficulty opening your eyes, or the sensation of pain when opening your eyes in the morning, can indicate an irritated eye from dryness or a type of corneal abrasion called an erosion. If the symptoms become severe, a more serious eye problem may be involved, such as a corneal ulcer or infection that needs to be treated immediately.

### Blurred Vision

It's common for patients with dry eye syndrome to have blurred or fluctuating vision much of the time; the lack of tears and the smooth optical surface they provide make focusing difficult. Blurry vision is frequently diagnosed as something other than dry eye, and doctors often prescribe tests looking for a brain tumor or stroke. Numerous patients have come to see me after having had computerized tomography (CT) or magnetic resonance imaging (MRI) that revealed nothing abnormal to explain the blurry vision. In virtually all these cases, it has turned out that the problem was caused by dry eye syndrome.

### Heavy or Tired Eyes

The feeling of heavy or tired eyes may result when the surface of the eye is not getting an adequate cleansing. Old, dirty tears containing allergens and irritants are not being properly removed from the ocular surface and replaced by healthy, fresh tears. As a result, the eyes may feel tired. It's like trying to wash windows with dirty dish water; the "window" never gets clean. Heavy eyes may also be caused by a situation called conjunctivochalasis, where the conjunctiva tissue is draped onto the lid margin.

### Excessively Watery Eyes

Ironically, dry eye syndrome can stimulate an overproduction of very watery tears. Normally, when a piece of dirt or other foreign body lodges in a healthy eye, the eye will produce lots of watery tears to wash the foreign body away. With chronic dry eye, the cornea may become so irritated that the same signal is sent to the tear glands, which then produce an abundance of watery tears. The cycle may keep repeating itself until the dry eye is properly treated.

### Excessive Mucus Discharge

Tears are made up of three layers: a watery layer, a fatty (lipid) layer, and a sugary protein or mucin layer. With some types of dry eye, the chemistry of the tear may be out of balance. The result is production of an excessive amount of mucus, which collects on the surface of the eye in little pieces or as a ropy strand.

### Sensitivity to Light

Dry eye sufferers very often experience significant pain in the presence of bright light, sunshine, or even fluorescent indoor lighting.

If you have all—or even some—of these symptoms and have been experiencing them for more than a week or two, you should consult with an eye doctor as soon as possible. However, before you do so, take the self-test in Box 1. It won't definitively diagnose you with dry eye syndrome (you need your doctor for that), but it can indicate if it's likely that you have this problem.

## WHO SUFFERS FROM DRY EYE SYNDROME?

According to the Schepens Eye Research Institute at Harvard University in Cambridge, Massachusetts, approximately 9 million Americans suffer from moderate to severe dry eye. (Other estimates go as high as 12 million!) Also, scientists estimate that an additional 20 to 30 million people may have mild cases of dry eye. However, a significant prevalence of dry eye occurs on other continents as well. Danish and Australian studies suggest that close to 10 percent of the adult European and Australian populations may have dry eye syndrome. A Japanese study showed that 33 percent of middle-aged adults have symptoms of dry eye. The condition seems to affect many more women than men (two to three times as many, according to Schepens), and its prevalence increases with age, becoming common among people over age 50.

The chances of developing dry eye syndrome increase if one or more of the following conditions or factors exists in your health history or everyday life; that is, if you:

Live in a very dry and/or windy region
Use a computer frequently
Use your eyes constantly for work or recreational activities, such as reading, watching television, or going to the movies
Frequently drive long distances
Smoke, or live with someone who smokes
Use medications for allergies, birth control, or depression
Take hormone replacement therapy
Have had cosmetic eye surgery, especially of the upper eyelids and/or the face
Have had LASIK eye surgery
Have worn contact lenses for many years
Suffer from certain illnesses, including Sjögren's syndrome, diabetes, thyroid disease, lupus, rheumatoid arthritis, osteoporosis, and ocular rosacea.

In many cases, dry eye syndrome can result from a combination of causes, such as thyroid disease coupled with menopause or the use of certain medications together with the prolonged wearing of contact lenses.

## TREATING DRY EYE

At this time the approach to treating dry eye is essentially the same whether you live in the United States, Europe, or another developed industrialized country. The standard initial treatment for mild to moderate dry eye is artificial tears, either an over-the-counter product or an individualized prescription. Or your doctor may elect to close your tear drains with a simple office procedure that keeps fresh tears on the eye longer. Also, a doctor may suggest a number of common home remedies. (All of these solutions will be discussed in detail later in the book.)

Severe dry eye, however, may lead to very serious eye problems, such as damage to the corneal epithelium, ulceration and infection of the cornea, and even severe visual impairment or blindness. Other forms of treatment are called for, including strong drugs or surgery. Again, if you are experiencing intractable dry eye symptoms, see an eye doctor as soon as possible.

## RECOMMENDED READING

At the present time, very little medical literature is available for the general reader on dry eye syndrome. In the Resources section at the back of this book, I've listed the professional literature I used to prepare this book. Two comprehensive books were especially useful to me. Although they are professional texts, both are clearly written. If you want additional information on any topic related to dry eye, I particularly recommend consulting these books: *Ocular Surface Disease: Medical and Surgical Management* by Edward J. Holland and Mark J. Mannis (eds.) and *Dry Eye and Ocular Surface Disorders* by Stephen C. Pflugfelder, Roger W. Beuerman, and Michael E. Stern (eds.).

BOX 1

## Do You Have Dry Eye Syndrome? A Self-Test

Answer "yes" or "no" to the following questions, and then read the commentary on each. If you answered affirmatively to one or more of the questions, you probably have at least a mild case of dry eye syndrome.

**1** *Do you have one or more of the symptoms of dry eye syndrome—scratching, stinging, pain, or redness in one or both eyes?*
If you are experiencing one or more of these symptoms and they do not respond within a day or two to over-the-counter artificial tears, don't ignore the symptoms or try further to self-treat. Call an eye doctor as soon as possible.

**2** *Have you had dry and irritated eyes for at least two weeks?*
If your eyes have been irritated for two weeks or longer, you've waited long enough. See an eye doctor as soon as possible. (If you don't already have an eye doctor, see Chapter 9 for instructions on how to locate and then screen a competent eye specialist.)

**3** *Is your eyesight constantly blurry and/or does the clarity of your vision fluctuate, even when you are wearing glasses or contact lenses?*
If you are experiencing blurry vision even when you are wearing your glasses or contacts, you may have a serious dry eye problem. If the vision fluctuates with blinking or improves when you use artificial tears, again the problem may be dry eye syndrome.

**4** *Have you been treating your eye problem with over-the-counter eyedrops or eye washes, but they have not solved your problem—or have made your problem worse?*

Most people try commercial eyedrops (artificial tears) when they first experience dry eye. Sometimes they help, although they're frequently inadequate for people with dry eye syndrome. If over-the-counter artificial tears don't seem to be easing your pain or are making your pain worse, stop using them. You may be allergic or sensitive to the preservatives in the drops. Again, see an eye doctor as soon as possible.

**5** *Do you spend most of your time in an office or home (or both) where the air is very dry? By the end of the day, are your eyes irritated?*
Sometimes the air in your work or home environment can irritate your eyes, especially if the air is too dry or too turbulent, as from a ceiling fan. Note if the air-conditioning or heating vents are aimed directly at or near your face; if so, take action to divert the air. Consider using a humidifier to moisten the air.

**6** *Do you work at a computer monitor or watch television for two or three hours without taking a break? Afterward, do your eyes hurt?*
Many people spend hour after hour working or playing in front of their computers without giving their eyes a much-needed rest. If you do this, you may already have, or may develop, a serious dry eye problem. Similar problems can develop among people who watch lots of television. At the very least, get up and walk around every thirty to forty-five minutes, use artificial tears, and blink your eyes frequently to lubricate them. If pain persists, call your doctor.

**7** *Have family members, friends, and coworkers started to ask you if there's something wrong with your eyes?*
If people are asking you if something is wrong with your eyes, the problem has now become prominent. Although

most people won't mention it, some may think that you've developed a problem with alcohol or drugs, which can also cause very red and irritated-looking eyes. Keep in mind that you could be giving an unfavorable impression of yourself with painfully bloodshot eyes.

**8** *Have you started taking a new medication (especially for allergy, depression, or hormone replacement therapy) and suddenly begun having problems with your eyes?*
Certain medications can cause dry eye problems. If you have chronic allergy problems, you may regularly take prescribed or over-the-counter medications, which can cause dry eye syndrome. Certain common prescription antidepressants can also cause dry eye. Other medications that can cause or contribute to dry eye syndrome include birth control pills, high blood pressure pills, and hormone replacement therapies.

**9** *Have you recently had LASIK surgery, but find that your eyes don't seem to be healing properly? Are your eyes scratchy and painful and is your vision somewhat blurry?*
If you've had LASIK surgery and your eyes are hurting after several weeks, it's possible that you have developed a dry eye problem. LASIK surgery is a very common cause of dry eye syndrome.

**10** *Do you need to wear sunglasses most of the time, even in the early evening or in dim light, to ease the pain from bright light?*
If you find that you're wearing sunglasses most of the time, both in and out of doors, you may have a potential dry eye problem. Sunlight or bright artificial light is possibly bothering you because of your severely dry eyes. If so, call an eye doctor for an evaluation.

CHAPTER

# 2

# An Overview of the Eye

Myth

*Dry eye syndrome is an isolated concern and has no impact on other eye disorders.*

Fact

*Vision disorders are layered phenomena, and treating dry eye effectively may not only improve comfort, but also help optimize vision when other problems exist.*

In order to better understand how dry eye develops and to comprehend what may be necessary in order to solve the problem, you need a basic course in eye anatomy. You probably learned all of this in high school biology class, but it's worth a quick review before moving on to the issues related to dry eye problems.

The human eye is frequently compared to a camera—so often, in fact, that the association is almost a cliché. However, like most clichés, the comparison is based in fact. Actually, it wouldn't surprise me if the inventor of the first camera used the anatomy of the eye as inspiration.

The camera and the eye work in much the same way. An image comes in through a lens and is recorded on some complex material at the back. In the camera, that material is film; in the eye, that material is the retina that in turn is connected to the optic nerve, which sends the image to the brain to interpret. (The inner layer of the retina actually leaves the back of the eye as the optic nerve. So, in effect, the retina is partly brain tissue.)

## PARTS OF THE EYE

Although the camera and the eye work in much the same way, the eye, not surprisingly, is a far more miraculous structure, made up of an incredible number of remarkably complex parts. Here is a quick description of these parts and a look at how they all work together.

### The Exterior Framework

The eye is much more than just the round globe that we think of as the "real eye." For starters, this globe, the eyeball, an extremely delicate structure, is located in what we sometimes call the eye socket, but what is formally known as the orbit. This cavity is formed at the juncture of three adjoining bones: the brow, the cheekbone, and the bridge of the nose. Working together, these tough bones support and protect the two delicate eyeballs. This bony shell is, of course, covered with skin.

Also present to protect the eyes are the eyelids. They appear to be simple flaps of skin, but in fact are also fascinating, complex structures. Eyelids are made up of tiny muscles (which allow the eye to open and close), blood vessels (which nourish the eyelid tissues), and glands (which produce tears). The purpose of the eyelids is to help keep the eye surface healthy and in satisfactory working condition, so that light and images can enter the eye without interruption to reach the retina and eventually the brain.

Like other complex organs in our bodies, under normal conditions the eyelids operate subconsciously, opening and shutting to help regulate light and protect the eyeballs from dirt or other foreign particles. They do this by blinking regularly, in

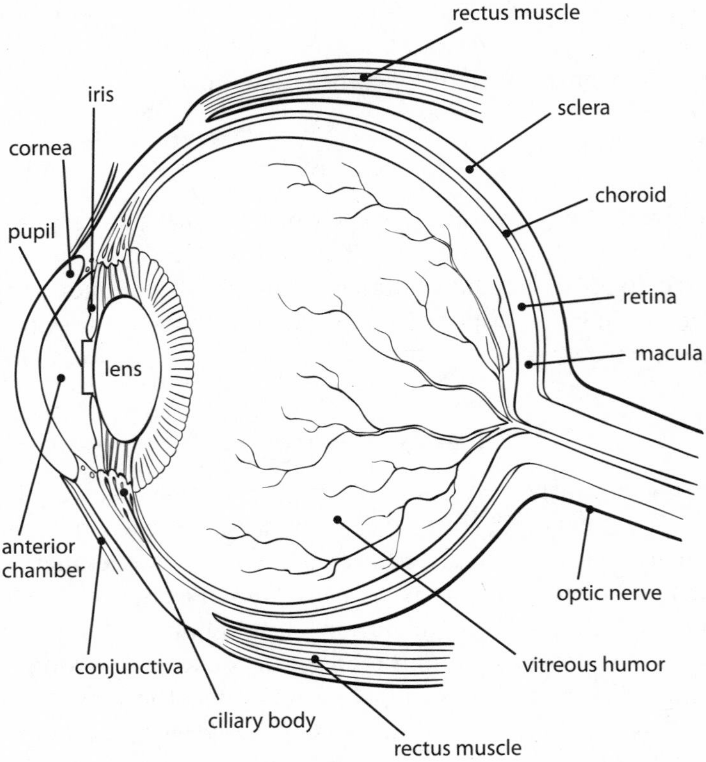


The Parts of the Eye.

order to distribute tears that lubricate and cleanse the surface of the eyes. The eyelids—and their various components—play a major role in the development and treatment of dry eye syndrome, and are discussed in greater detail in Chapter 3.

In addition to the tiny muscles within the eyelids, several other muscles surround the eyeballs and are attached to the sclera, or outside covering of the eyeballs. These muscles are synchronized and allow the two eyes to move in concert, left and right, up and down.

BOX 2

**Not Just for Looks!**

Eyebrows, the thin bits of wispy hair that cover the bony brow, and eyelashes, the fringe of hairs on the edges of the eyelids, do not exist merely for the sake of beauty—they are hardworking features designed to protect the eyes. Both brows and lashes catch airborne flying matter before it can reach (and possibly damage) the cornea, and eyebrows also serve to direct perspiration away from the eyes. Despite what cosmetic experts may say, eyebrows and eyelashes are much more than elements to be shaped, plucked, colored, and curled to make you look better, they are important tools present to ensure eye health.

## The Eyeball

The eyeball is made up of many layers of tissue. The *conjunctiva* is a transparent membrane that lines the inner eyelid and covers the front of the eyeball, except for the cornea. It is attached to the *sclera,* the dense white tissue often referred to as the "white of the eyes" that is essentially the eye wall. The conjunctiva is a wet, mucosal surface, like the lining of the mouth or the nose. It contains cells (known as goblet cells because of their wine-goblet shape) that secrete a mucus-like substance called *mucin,* which ultimately forms the inner layer of the tear. The conjunctiva also contains tiny blood vessels that not only nourish these important cells, but also provide access to the surface of the eye for the white blood cells, the universal protector of living tissue. Between the conjunctiva and the sclera is a layer of connective tissue called the episclera.

At the center of the eye is the *cornea,* or what some people refer to as the window of the eye. The cornea is divided into three major sections: the outer surface epithelium, which accounts for about 10 percent of the entire thickness; the stroma, which accounts for almost 90 percent of the cornea thickness; and the endothelium, a single layer of cells lining the inner cornea, which keeps the stroma from swelling by removing excess water. The cornea is surrounded by the conjunctiva and is transparent.

The area where the cornea and conjunctiva connect (for "geographical purposes," this is where the white part meets the colored part of the eye) is a several-millimeter-wide zone of stem cells. The cornea, like skin, regularly sloughs off dead surface epithelial cells. The cornea's stem cells, located in the peripheral edge of the cornea, replace older, degenerate cells of the central cornea. When severe dry eye develops, the cornea's stem cell activity can be dangerously affected; this extremely serious situation can lead to altered vision, with scarring of the cornea and possibly blindness.

The cornea allows light to enter the eye and, working together with the lens, permits the eye to focus. Behind the cornea and in front of the lens are the *pupil* and the *iris* (the membrane that gives your eye its color—blue, brown, or hazel). The pupil is the black "dot" at the center of the colored iris, although actually it is the hole through which light passes from the eye to the retina. To return to our camera simile, the iris acts like the aperture of a camera, constricting in bright light and dilating in dim light, and thus controlling the amount of light that passes through.

Between the cornea and the iris lies the *anterior chamber.* This space is filled with *aqueous humor,* a transparent fluid that nourishes the cells inside the eye. The fluid is manufactured in the posterior chamber of the eye, by the ciliary body located behind the attachment of the iris.

Behind the iris in the posterior chamber is the *lens.* This clear, colorless, normally elastic tissue is enclosed in a capsule and suspended in the middle of the eye by a net of support fibers. The lens changes shape in order to focus light rays on the retina. When an object is close up, the lens thickens in order to

BOX 3

**Floaters**

No doubt from time to time you have noticed dark-colored bits and pieces floating around in your field of vision. Strangely enough, even by doctors, these floating pieces are called simply floaters. They are actually leftover cellular debris from the maturation and breakdown of the vitreous humor in front of the retina. Normally floaters are of no concern, but if you suddenly become aware of new floaters, especially if they are accompanied by flashes of light or unusual curtain-like images or shadows, see your eye doctor immediately. Sometimes floaters can indicate a more serious situation, such as a retinal tear or detachment.

best perceive the image. When an object is farther away, the lens thins out in order to focus on the object more clearly.

Behind the lens is a large, round area known as the *vitreous chamber,* which makes the "ball" of the eyeball. It is filled with a gelatinous liquid known as the *vitreous humor.*

At the back of the vitreous chamber is the *retina.* To return to the camera image, the retina of the eye is comparable to film in the camera, in that it "processes" the light projected through the cornea and the lens. Amazingly, the retina is composed of ten layers. Among them are special cells known as rod cells (which respond to light) and cone cells (which respond to color and transform light into electrical impulses, which enable the visual signal to travel along the optic nerve to the brain). Rod cells outnumber cone cells 20-to-1. Also, cone cells need more light to function, which is (in part) why it is difficult to see colors in the dark.

At the center of the retina is a small depression known as the fovea. Made up only of cone cells, it is the most visually sensitive part of the eye. The area immediately surrounding the fovea, known as the macula lutea, is responsible for central vision, or the vision that you use in order to look directly at something, as opposed to peripheral vision.

### From the Eye to the Brain

The retina is nourished primarily by the choroid, a multilayered tissue composed of veins and arteries which lies between the retina and the posterior sclera. (By the way, the sclera, the white tissue that surrounds the iris, extends around the entire eyeball.)

The *optic nerve* leaves the eye on its journey to the brain at a structure called the optic disc. This part of the optic nerve is the only section that can be readily examined in the office by your doctor. It can reveal important information with regard to glaucoma, diabetes, and other eye diseases and disorders.

The optic nerve takes the electrical impulses recorded by the retina and transmits them to the visual cortex at the back of the brain, where the impulses are interpreted.

## WHEN YOUR EYES WORK WELL

Despite this long list of eye parts, the ultimate act of "seeing" is relatively simple. As with the camera, light is projected through the cornea, the pupil, and the lens. The internal eye muscles adjust the shape of the lens to focus the light rays onto the retina. There the rods and cones turn the light into electrical impulses that are carried by the optic nerve to the brain.

The image received by the retina is upside down, characteristic of a simple convex lens. As a result, when the impulse moves on to the brain, the brain takes this image and turns it right side up. The brain also coordinates the images from the two eyes, which are slightly different, merging the two to produce three-dimensional vision.

That's it—the phenomenon of vision!

## EYE PROBLEMS: AN OVERVIEW

Not surprisingly, given that the eye is such a complex organ, a host of problems can arise that involve the health of your eyes and/or your vision. Many of these problems have little or nothing to do with dry eye syndrome—although some are directly relevant. It is helpful to become acquainted with a few of the more common ailments, and to understand how best to deal with them.

### Refraction Problems

The common problems of nearsightedness, farsightedness, astigmatism, and presbyopia—those issues that force us to wear glasses or contact lenses—are what are known as refraction problems. Refraction problems result from errors in how the lens and cornea transmit images in one or both eyes. When light rays come through your eye, the cornea and the lens bend (refract) them. For the image to be clear, the lens, cornea, and length of the eyeball must be properly coordinated. When they are not, the image that reaches the retina is not in focus.

*Nearsightedness,* also known as myopia, results when light is focused in front of the retina, and only objects at close range are in focus. To put it another way, most people who are nearsighted have eyeballs that are slightly elongated, so that light rays fail to reach the retina. Occasionally, nearsightedness can be caused by a "steep" cornea or lens that bends incoming light too sharply in view of the distance to the retina.

The most common treatment for nearsightedness is corrective glasses or contact lenses. However, an increasingly popular solution is LASIK or other refractive surgery. LASIK is a surgical technique in which the cornea is flattened, thereby reducing the bending of light on its journey to the retina. Unfortunately, many people who have had LASIK surgery develop dry eye (see Chapter 8).

*Farsightedness* results when light is focused on the retina

BOX 4

**Time for Granny Glasses**

Ever wonder why everyone seems to need reading glasses after they turn 40? Well, here's the reason. The lens of the eye is composed of cell fibers. As we age, the lens accumulates more and more fibers that ultimately makes it less elastic. The rigid lens creates a problem known as presbyopia. By middle age, we are less able to focus on close-up objects such as the morning paper, the telephone book, and grocery labels.

The traditional solution is reading glasses. In fact, many nearsighted people, when they reach middle age, discover that they must wear bifocals or trifocals, reading glasses, or even reading glasses over their contact lenses to accommodate both their nearsightedness and their presbyopia.

from objects only at long range, usually because the eyeball is too short from back to front. Thus, the rays of light converge beyond the retina, or beyond the length at which they would be in focus. As with nearsightedness, the condition can also be caused by problems with the lens and the cornea. Farsightedness can be easily treated with eyeglasses or contact lenses.

*Astigmatism* results from an uneven curvature of the cornea. A normal cornea is symmetrical, whereas with astigmatism the cornea has areas that are steep, bumpy, or flattened like a football rather than round like a basketball. Astigmatism often accompanies nearsightedness or farsightedness. It usually can be treated with eyeglasses or contact lenses.

*Presbyopia* occurs when the lens of the eye becomes less elastic and is therefore less able to bring material at close range into focus. This "hardening" of the lens is a natural part of aging, becoming noticeable around age 40, and happens to most people to some extent. It can be treated with eyeglasses. The problem tends to worsen until about age 65, requiring people to have their "reading" prescription changed every few years. However, by age 65 the lens of the eye has lost virtually all of its elasticity and the level of presbyopia stabilizes.

### Injury or Trauma to the Eye

Especially because it is so delicate, the eye can be injured relatively easily. Trauma can result from the presence of foreign bodies, chemical or ultraviolet burns, or blows to the eye.

If a foreign body (dust, dirt, an eyelash) lodges in your eye, you will immediately feel sharp pain, start blinking repeatedly, and tears will naturally flow, sometimes washing out the offending object. At other times the foreign object may be more problematic (a sliver of wood or a piece of glass) and the natural "washing" is not enough to solve the problem. The foreign body may actually perforate the eyeball and lodge inside! When this occurs, go to a hospital emergency room or see an ophthalmologist immediately. Don't try to remove the object yourself; you can cause additional pain and injury to the eye. Your doctor may need to remove the object surgically, or, if the offending object is gone and only your cornea is scratched, he or she may just treat it with antibiotic drops until it is healed.

Chemical burns result when a potent chemical substance such as bleach, ammonia, lye, or some other toxin comes in contact with the surface of the eye—often with a casual splash. The eye can also be burned by ultraviolet rays, such as light from arc welding or the reflection of light off snow. Chemical and ultraviolet burns cause severe pain, hypersensitivity to light, and possibly even permanent loss of vision.

If your eye is burned by a chemical, flush it out immediately with clear water and continue doing so for at least thirty minutes. Then go to a hospital emergency room or an ophthalmologist immediately. Depending on the seriousness of the injury, your eye may need additional attention to promote healing. If the conjunctiva, cornea, or eyelid is severely damaged, it may require surgery.

Black eye may result from blunt trauma to the eye caused by an accident or fight. A black eye consists of broken conjunctival blood vessels over the white of the eye, and swelling with dislocation of the lid and tissue around the eye. While in some cases a black eye, because of the bruising, may look worse than it actually is and will clear in a week or two, it is wise to have the eye checked by an eye doctor within twenty-four hours to make sure the eyeball has not been seriously damaged.

Like black eye, hyphema usually results from blunt trauma to the eye and is characterized by bleeding in the anterior chamber. Hyphema may also originate from severe inflammation of the iris, a blood vessel abnormality, or a growth within the eye itself. See an eye doctor within twenty-four hours.

## Common Eyelid Disorders

The eyelid, and particularly the glands contained within the eyelid, play a pivotal role in the development of dry eye. (The anatomy and physiology is explained in Chapter 3.) A number of common disorders can show up on the eyelid, some of which relate directly to dry eye, and it is helpful to know a bit about them.

A sty (or acute hordeolum) is an acute, usually noninfected inflammatory condition that forms owing to an obstruction at the opening of a meibomian gland, behind the root of an eyelash. It is characterized by painful swelling on the eyelid margin, and possibly blurred vision from pressure on the cornea. It usually develops gradually, forming a painful red lump that sometimes has a white head which, after several days, may disappear.

A chalazion is a chronic form of swelling on the eyelid, which results from a blockage of one of the meibomian glands.

While a sty is painful, a chalazion is usually painless and may disappear within a few weeks; if it does not, see an eye doctor.

Blepharitis is an inflammation of the eyelid edges that may produce the sensation that a foreign object is in the eye. The eye and the eyelid may itch and burn, the edge of the eyelid may become red, and the eye may become watery and sensitive to bright light. The eyelid may swell and some of the eyelashes may fall out.

Blepharitis can develop as one of two types: anterior or posterior. Anterior blepharitis is typically caused by microbes such as bacteria or parasites such as mites, and is characterized by a scaling or crusting around the lashes and lid margin. Sometimes small pockets of inflammation develop at the base of the eyelashes and form shallow ulcers, a condition known as ulcerative blepharitis. During sleep, the eyelids may become "glued" shut.

Posterior blepharitis develops because of abnormal meibomian gland function, which can cause lid inflammation and lipid tear deficiency or both. Posterior blepharitis is closely associated with dry eye syndrome, and is discussed in greater detail in Chapter 4.

Sties, chalazions, and blepharitis are all inflammatory in nature. Other eyelid disorders may involve the abnormal positioning of the eyelid.

Ptosis, or drooping eyelid, usually results from a weakness of the muscle responsible for raising the lid. This can be a congenital problem (that may require surgery), or it can result from weakening muscles due to aging. It can also be caused by diseases such as myasthenia gravis, stroke, or diabetes.

Entropion is a condition in which the upper or lower eyelid turns in, allowing the lashes to scratch the eye. In severe cases, an ulcerating or scarring can occur on the cornea. Ectropion is the reverse situation; the lower lid turns out, causing tears to flow out of the eye instead of lubricating the eye. These problems usually are part of the aging process, but they can also result from underlying conditions such as atopic dermatitis or lupus erythematosus.

## Common Eyeball Disorders

Conjunctivitis, commonly known as pink eye, is an inflammation of the conjunctiva, the transparent membrane that lines the eyelid and the eyeball up to the margin of the cornea. Conjunctivitis can be caused by a bacterial or a viral infection, an allergic or toxic reaction, a clogged tear duct, or dry eye syndrome. It may be characterized by redness, a gritty feeling in the eye, itching, and a discharge that can form a crust while sleeping. It can also cause blurred vision and sensitivity to light. Conjunctivitis may also be caused by inadequate hygiene; for example, giant papillary or contact lens–related conjunctivitis is frequently caused by wearing inadequately cleaned contact lenses.

Scleritis and episcleritis are characterized by inflammation of the sclera or the episclera. These problems are often associated with systemic disease, such as rheumatoid arthritis or lupus.

Keratitis is an inflammation of the cornea and can be very serious. The cornea is possibly the most vulnerable part of the eye. It can be easily injured or can become inflamed by the presence of foreign objects or by being burned by the sun or ultraviolet light. Sometimes the injury can become infected and ulcers can develop. Even problems in other parts of the eye, such as blepharitis, can harm the cornea.

## Serious Vision Disorders

Many of the diseases and disorders of the eye come into play as we age, and many are inherited. Most important, many of these diseases can lead to blindness if not treated promptly and properly. Among the better-known serious vision disorders are cataract, glaucoma, macular degeneration, and detached retina.

*Cataract* is the most common eye disorder among the elderly; almost all people over age 60 have varying stages of cataract formation. Cataract can be related to other diseases such as diabetes.

A cataract is a clouding of the lens of the eye, which, when healthy, is clear. Symptoms include blurred vision, impaired vision at night or in bright light, and halos around lights. Cataract is one of the easiest eye problems to treat because today's sophisticated surgery can restore sight virtually completely.

*Glaucoma* is actually a group of diseases of the eye with one common feature: progressive damage to the optic nerve due to excessive pressure within the eyeball. As the optic nerve deteriorates, blind spots and patterns develop. Left untreated, glaucoma can cause total blindness.

Glaucoma has two forms, acute and chronic. The latter is, by far, the more common. Both types occur more commonly among elderly, farsighted people. Acute glaucoma develops quickly and is characterized by blurred vision (usually in one eye), halos around lights, severe pain in the eye, and redness. Chronic glaucoma, which is characterized by the gradual loss of peripheral vision, is perhaps more frightening because it can go undetected for years, then escalate very quickly. Special tests can be given to detect early stages of glaucoma.

*Macular degeneration* is another disease most commonly seen among the elderly. Deposits may form and blood vessels may grow in the macular region between the retina and its supporting layer of choroid tissue. (The macula marks the central point of the retina and is responsible for central vision.) These deposits and vessels can cause serious impairment of central vision, although peripheral vision is not affected. During early stages of the problem, the leaking blood vessels can be treated with laser therapy. Patients with macular degeneration should be seen by an eye doctor trained in retina diseases (Chapter 9).

*Retinal detachment,* as its name suggests, results when the retina develops a tear or a hole, usually the result of trauma or aging. With retinal detachment, the vitreous humor leaks through the tear and under the retina to lift it away from the underlying layer. Symptoms may include flashing sensations, floaters, blurred vision, and a shadow over a portion of the field of vision. If your retina becomes detached, it can usually be repaired through surgery. If a tear or hole has not yet resulted in detachment, laser or freezing (cryo treatment) can prevent detachment.

You now have a basic working knowledge of the anatomy of the eye, and an overview of the problems that may affect your eyes and your vision. Some of these problems are closely related to dry eye syndrome. We need now to look at dry eye in detail, and then view its causes.

CHAPTER

# 3

# The Dry Eye

Myth

*Tears are vestigial fluids left over from prehistoric times and serve no particular purpose except to show emotion.*

Fact

*Tears are as essential to the health of the eye as blood is to the internal organs.*

Tears perform a number of functions. Working together with the eyelids, tears protect, cleanse, and nourish the eye. In one way like miniature wipers, the eyelids distribute tears over the eyes, clearing off and flushing away dust, dirt, everyday debris, and—most important—bacteria and other potential disease-causing agents. In addition, they transport proteins, vitamins, and other important nutrients onto the eyes, where they are absorbed into the cornea. Tears also lubricate the eyeballs and prevent dehydration of conjunctival mucus membranes and other tissues associated with the eyes. Finally, when all is working well, tears create a smooth optical surface on the cornea and ensure that a high-quality image can be projected onto the retina.

Dry eye syndrome, to a great extent, develops when systems in the eyelids and the various tear glands go haywire. In order to begin to understand dry eye, we need to take a closer look at the anatomy and physiology of the eyelids and the tear glands that are responsible for the production of our precious tears.

## HUMAN EYELIDS

Human eyelids are amazing little structures. Although thin and delicate, they are actually complex, powerful mechanisms containing an intricate collection of muscles, nerves, blood vessels, and glands that act as the first line of defense against injury to the eye. They respond quickly and forcefully when a foreign body threatens the eye. While we are awake, our eyelids open and shut, or blink, about once every seven seconds, sweeping precious tears over the eyeballs to keep them moist. While we are asleep, the eyelids close over the eyes, shielding and protecting them from airborne foreign bodies and even the soft pillowcase that may accidentally touch (and possibly harm!) our eyes as we turn during the night. Blinking is usually an involuntary reflex, invoked subconsciously, not unlike the way our hearts keep pounding without our thinking about it. Unlike the beating of the heart, we can choose to override the blink reflex and control it to some extent. Our eyelids also contain some of the glands that help create the valuable liquid known as tears. (Actually, additional glands outside the eyelid are the primary tear producers, but more about that shortly.)

## TEAR GLANDS

In general, a gland is a cell, a group of cells, or an organ that selectively removes material from the blood, concentrates or alters it as necessary, secretes it for further use, or eliminates it from the body. Tear glands are the glandular organs that perform these functions with regard to our eyes.

Dry eye syndrome can manifest itself in a number of ways, but it almost always results from some sort of disruption of the tear glands. For example, excessively dry eyes may be due to inadequate tear production, the type of dry eye known as aqueous tear deficient dry eye. Here the lacrimal glands do not produce enough tears to maintain adequate lubrication of the conjunctiva and cornea. Or dry eye may result from an abnormal tear composition that causes overly rapid evaporation of the tears, a form known as *evaporative dry eye*. With this type, although the lacrimal glands produce sufficient watery tears, the meibomian glands do not supply enough lipid. Thus the evaporation is so quick that the conjunctiva and cornea cannot be kept adequately covered with a layer of tears.

## The Lacrimal System

The *lacrimal glands* are part of what is known as the lacrimal system or the lacrimal apparatus, comprising a complex of lacrimal glands that produce aqueous (watery) tears and ducts that allow "old" or "dirty" tears to drain from the eyes. The large main lacrimal gland is found under the upper eyelid, toward the side of the eye near the ear. Smaller accessory lacrimal glands are mostly situated next to the main lacrimal gland in the crease of the lining of the upper lid and the eyeball.

At the marginal edge of the inner corner of the upper and lower lids, next to the nose, are two small holes known as the upper and lower puncta, which serve as portals for draining away old tears into a duct system that includes the lacrimal canaliculi, a lacrimal sac, and ultimately the lacrimal duct, which drains the tears into the nose.

When the lacrimal glands fail to produce enough watery tears, aqueous tear deficient dry eye can develop.

## The Meibomian Glands

*Meibomian glands* are lipid (oil)-secreting glands that are embedded in the upper and lower eyelids. The upper eyelid has thirty to forty individual meibomian glands, the lower lid has twenty to twenty-five, and in both cases the glands are lined up in a single row perpendicular to the upper and lower eyelid margins.

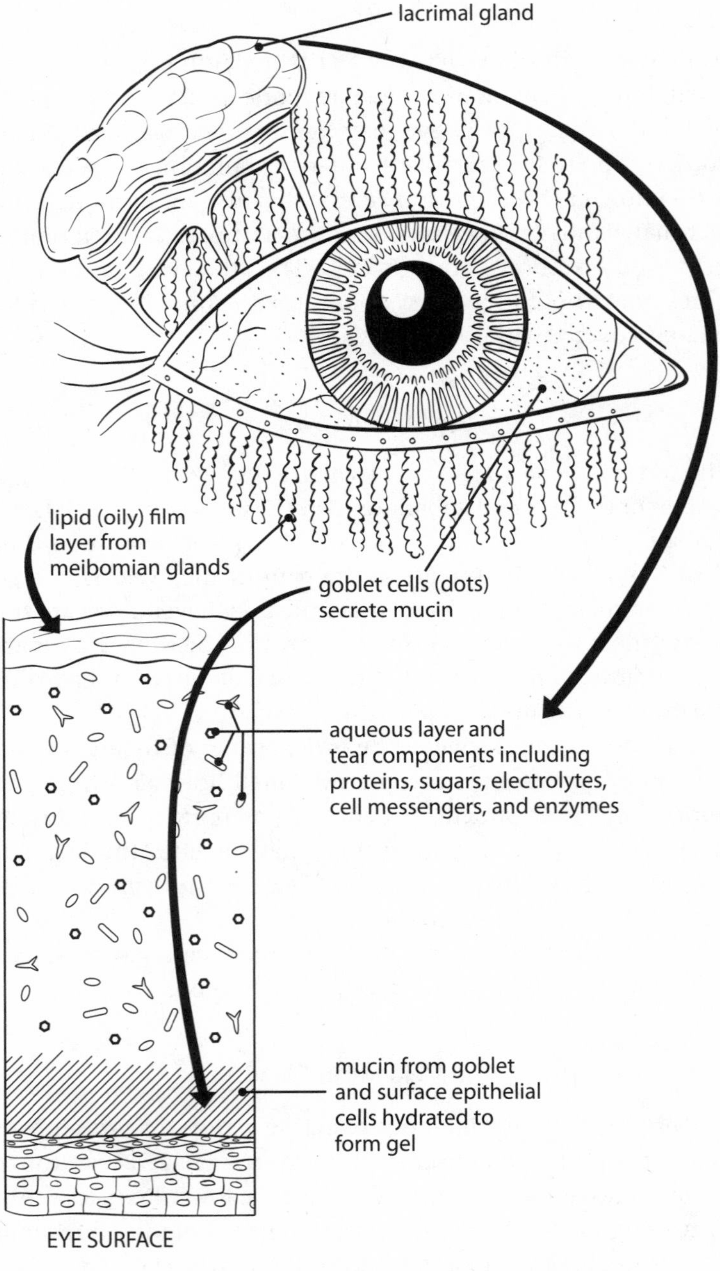


The Tear System. At lower left is a cross-section of tear film.

Each meibomian gland comprises many tiny sacs called acini, which are interconnected by a long central common duct running the length of the gland. Cells that make up the acini synthesize the meibomian gland lipids and release them into the central gland duct. These lipids are then excreted as an oily substance called meibum, which consists mostly of liquid wax, cholesterol-related molecules, and other lipids. The meibum is secreted onto the ocular surface through the gland orifice located at the lid margin just behind the eyelash, where it joins with the aqueous water to create the tear film.

When the meibomian glands fail to produce lipid properly, the resulting condition, known as meibomian gland dysfunction (or posterior blepharitis), can lead to evaporative dry eye.

### Mucin-Producing Cells

In addition to the tear glands, certain cells, called goblet epithelial cells, which are found in the conjunctiva, produce a glycoprotein (or carbohydrate/protein) substance called *mucin,* which is vital to the makeup of tears. (Mucin is also produced by the cornea's epithelial cells.) Disturbances in the production of mucin can ultimately lead to dry eye. Mucin-producing disturbances can be caused by inflammation or infection of the conjunctiva, chemical burns, trauma, and even malnutrition (specifically a vitamin-A deficiency called xerophthalmia). In these situations the conjunctiva becomes abnormally dry and the cornea becomes "nonwettable"; in other words, water (or the aqueous tears) will not adhere properly to the surface of the eye.

## TEAR FILM

Until now, you may have thought that tears were simply wet, salty waterworks that appeared when you were very sad, joyously happy, or suffering from a bad cold. Not so. Tears are not only a complex, delicately balanced brew, but are fundamental to a healthy, functional eye. Also, of course, tears are a pivotal factor with regard to the development of dry eye.

## Three Important Layers

The moist substance that coats our eyes at all times—known as tear film—consists of three layers: the lipid layer, the aqueous layer, and the mucin layer.

The lipid layer is the oily, outer layer of the tear film and is made up of the waxy meibum produced by the meibomian glands. The lipid layer serves a number of important purposes. It provides protection for the eye from microbes in the air and undesirable skin oils. It also forms a hydrophobic barrier that prevents tears from overflowing onto the lids, and it creates a seal that keeps our eyes lubricated while we sleep. Most important, the lipid layer helps reduce tear evaporation during our waking hours.

The aqueous layer is the middle and thickest layer of the tear film. Since it is made up mostly of water, it serves as a rinsing agent for irritants such as dust and dirt. It also helps dilute noxious agents, such as infectious microbes, topical medications, and allergens.

Secreted by the lacrimal glands, the aqueous layer, in addition to water, contains a complex collection of proteins, electrolytes, and antibodies and other secretions that help keep the eye healthy and free from infection. One example is lysozyme, a highly effective antibacterial agent. Lysozyme attacks and inactivates bacteria on the surface of the eye in a matter of minutes. Without it and other microbe-fighting secretions, our eyes would be prey to disease, and eye infections would be rampant.

The mucin layer is the innermost layer of the tear film, the layer that attaches to the surface of the eye. It is made up of the mucins, the glycoproteins produced by goblet cells in the conjunctiva and in the cornea's epithelial cells. The mucin layer serves two functions. First, because of its mucousy texture, it allows the tear film to attach to the cornea and thus helps to spread tears evenly across the surface of the eye. Second, it stabilizes the tear film by creating a hydrated gel matrix that allows the water from the aqueous layer to moisten and nourish the cornea. Both of these functions lengthen what is called tear breakup time (TBUT)—the time it takes for the tear film to become unstable and nonwettable after it is exposed to the air—which further protects the eye.

This trilayered tear film is absolutely essential to the overall health of the eye. If one component is not doing its job, the tear film will destabilize more rapidly than it should; as a result, the ocular surface is exposed. Prolonged or repeated exposure creates symptoms of dry eye (what is sometimes called mild dry eye) and may ultimately damage the corneal epithelium. If the dry eye symptoms are addressed and adequate lubrication is provided, the damaged epithelium will repair itself nicely; however, if the dry eye symptoms are not treated, the epithelium will continue to break down.

## THE PRODUCTION OF HEALTHY TEARS

Tears are produced as part of a system that some experts refer to as the lacrimal functional unit. This unit or system is made up of the ocular surface (including the cornea, the conjunctiva, and its mucin-producing goblet cells), the meibomian glands, the lacrimal glands, the eyelids, and the network of nerves that connects them. Acting through areas of the central nervous system, a complex of sensory, autonomic (involuntary), and motor (voluntary) nerves links the components of the lacrimal functional unit into a loop. These components work together to allow the eye surface to maintain a sense of equilibrium and health.

The system has four active parts: the incoming message, the outgoing command, tear secretion, and the blink.

### The Incoming Message

The surface of the eye (including the cornea and the conjunctiva) is covered with sensory nerves. In fact, the cornea alone has a density of free nerve endings at least twenty times that of tooth pulp. The incoming message occurs when a foreign body (such

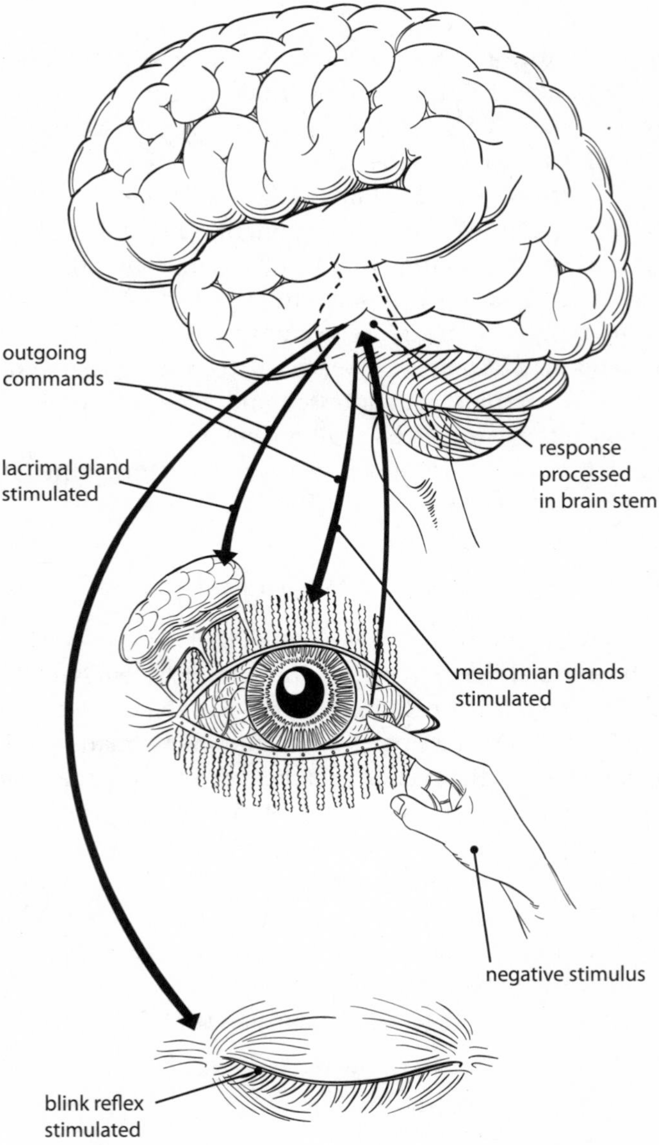


The Lacrimal Functional Unit.

as an eyelash, a piece of dust or dirt, an allergen, or a toxin) stimulates the nerves on the surface of the eye, and the nerves send a message to the brain stem. The incoming message can also be activated by emotional stimulation, which is processed differently by the brain but still instigates the tear-producing process.

### The Outgoing Command

When the brain receives the message from the surface of the eye, it processes the information and sends a command to the lacrimal glands to secrete aqueous tears. The meibomian glands and mucin-producing goblet cells may receive similar orders from the nervous system to produce meibum and mucin, respectively. In addition, the brain sends a message to the eyelid muscles, stimulating the blink mechanism.

### Tear Secretion

When the tear glands receive their orders, they secrete their respective substances (aqueous, meibum, and mucin), which in turn combine on the surface of the eyes as tears.

### The Blink

Like the tear-gland secretions, blinking may be induced by stimulation to the ocular surface. When the eyelid muscles receive their command, they blink.

Blinking can be both involuntary and voluntary. Normal blinking is involuntary, but we can override it and control the blink process. The actual stimulus responsible for a basic, involuntary blink has not been identified, although recent studies suggest that it may be the change in temperature that occurs with the breakdown of the tear film on the surface of the eye.

Healthy involuntary blinking occurs about every seven seconds. With a normal blink, the eyes close more or less from the temporal, or outer, side of the eye to the nasal side, distributing fresh tears over the ocular surface. The tears are pushed toward and pumped into the puncta at the inner corner of the eye and are drained into the nasolacrimal sac within the nose.

### Closing the Loop

The tear secretion and blinking of the eye in effect close the loop of the lacrimal functional unit, and the process starts all over again. The tear film begins to evaporate; the exposed nerves send a message to the brain; the brain sends a command to the tear glands to secrete and to the eyelids to blink; and, once again, the tears are secreted and the blink distributes them. The creation and distribution of tears is, of necessity, a dynamic process because in order to maintain the health of the ocular surface, the tears must be continually cleared and replaced.

The rate of removal of newly produced tears is called *tear clearance*. It is regulated by the rate of the production of new tear components, the redistribution of tears onto the ocular surface through the action of blinking, and the rate of drainage of old tears into the nasolacrimal sac.

## WHEN TEARS DRY UP

Dry eye syndrome is more than simply the lack of sufficient tears. Instability of the tear film makeup or disruption of any facet of the tear production or distribution system can lead to dry eye syndrome or more serious eye problems. Specifically, tear production can break down in several ways, as described below.

### Insufficient Watery Tears

Insufficient production of watery tears, a common cause of dry eye syndrome, indicates a disruption in the lacrimal gland system; in other words, the lacrimal glands are not producing enough aqueous tears. Lack of watery tears has a profound effect

BOX 5

## Crocodile Tears

The fake watery displays put on by children when, for example, they are told they can't have an ice cream cone, have been of interest to scientists for hundreds of years. In truth, the concept of crocodile tears does refer to the supposed behavior of crocodiles: specifically, when crocodiles stalk, kill, and eat their prey, they are thought to weep. This belief has led to the notion that feigned sorrow in humans is expressed symbolically as "crocodile tears."

Like humans, crocodiles possess lacrimal glands that produce watery tears. However, these tears are not shed onto the ocular surface, but instead flow directly into the nasobuccal (nose-mouth) cavity of the crocodile, possibly to lubricate his food. Thus, when a crocodile looks like he's weeping as he eats, his glands are simply secreting tears (instead of saliva) into his gigantic mouth.

Humans may, at times, exhibit a similar type of medically based crocodile tears, in that they sometimes shed tears while tasting or chewing food. This phenomenon results from misdirected messages to the lacrimal glands, usually from injured facial nerves. Often this misguided signal is given in only one eye, while the unaffected eye sheds normal tears.

The expression "crocodile tears" showed up in another context in the 1950s, as the result of a procedure developed by Russian and Chinese doctors for the treatment of dry eye. After the procedure, the saliva of the patients overflowed into their lower lids, creating supposed tears that were referred to as "crocodile tears." Although the procedure soothed dry eye symptoms, it was later abandoned, perhaps because of its rather disconcerting side effects.

Today, although children may still succeed in manipulating their parents with hypocritical crocodile tears, it seems unlikely that real crocodiles are doing anything more than digesting their prey when they appear to be weeping over their dinner.

BOX 6

**Why Onions Make You Cry**

When onions are cut up, they release a chemical into the air that turns into a sulfuric compound when it makes contact with the surface of your eye. Left to its own devices, this sulfuric compound can cause extreme damage to the cornea, not to mention incredible pain. But when the onion chemical reaches the surface of the eye, nerves in the cornea trigger the lacrimal glands to secrete watery tears, which dilute the chemical, making it harmless. In other words, we begin to "cry."

Even though we're naturally protected, nobody really likes tearing up while chopping onions. To prevent crying, try these remedies: Place your onions in the freezer for five or six minutes before slicing them; wash the onions in cool water before chopping; squirt a few drops of lemon juice on the onion just after you cut into it; leave the root end intact while cutting; or place a lighted candle near you as you slice or chop. Perhaps these suggestions will help keep those onion-chopping crying jags to a minimum!

on the eye. Specifically, a lack of watery tears results in an increase in saltiness on the ocular surface. In turn, the increased saltiness damages the epithelial layer of the cornea and the conjunctiva, causing certain enzymes to be released and an inflammatory reaction to occur. This reaction further disrupts lacrimal gland function and causes further erosion to the surface of the tissues, which creates a vicious cycle.

Paradoxically, dry eye syndrome can be characterized by the production of too many tears. This happens when the surface of the eye becomes so dry and irritated that excess tears are stimulated and produced as a reflex in response to the irritated ocular surface.

### Insufficient Lipids

Insufficient lipids indicate a disruption in the meibomian gland system. As a result, the lipid outer layer of the tear film is abnormal and tears evaporate too quickly with increased saltiness. As with insufficient watery tears, the result is inflammation and further disruption of the tear gland function with increased dryness and corneal and conjunctival erosion.

### Insufficient Mucin

Lack of sufficient mucin will also generate instability of the tear film. As we've seen, insufficient mucin can result from inflammation or infection of the conjunctiva, chemical burns, trauma, and even malnutrition. Although it is far less common than the other causes, it too can lead to dry eye.

## BREAKDOWN OF THE LACRIMAL FUNCTIONAL UNIT

The four-part lacrimal functional unit can go awry for a number of reasons. For example, the incoming message can be disrupted if the surface of the eye has been traumatized or numbed in any way. The command from the brain to the glands and eyelids can be short-circuited, often as a result of certain diseases. Finally, the secretion of tears and the blink can be disrupted if the message or the command has been muted or shut down, if the tear glands are diseased, or if the eyelid muscles are disabled.

So, what *causes* these disruptions? The answer is complicated and multifaceted, but important to understand if you suffer from dry eye. We look at it in detail in the next chapter.

CHAPTER

# 4

# The Causes

Myth

*Dry eye is caused simply by reduced tear production.*

Fact

*Dry eye is a complex syndrome caused by inadequate tear production, secretion, or distribution, and often may be associated with serious systemic diseases, including Sjögren's syndrome, lupus, and diabetes.*

Dry eye is a syndrome. By definition, a syndrome is an abnormality characterized by a group of signs and symptoms that often occur simultaneously. We've seen that dry eye manifests as mild to extreme dryness of the cornea (the clear "window" at the front of the eye) and the conjunctiva (the mucus membrane that covers the eyeball, excluding the cornea, as well as the lining of the eyelid). This dryness is due to inadequate tear production, increased tear evaporation, or both. The symptoms may include a constant sense of itchiness, scratchiness, or grittiness; the feeling of a foreign object in the eyes; burning or stinging; chronic redness or inflammation of the conjunctiva (making the whites of the eyes appear red); a sharp sensitivity to light; varying degrees of pain, even extreme pain; and fluctuating vision. And yes, sometimes dry eye can even cause your eyes to tear excessively!

What exactly causes our tear secretion system to break down?

Like the symptoms, the causes of dry eye syndrome are numerous and varied. In grossly general terms, dry eye syndrome is caused by a number of very disparate problems. These include:

Behavioral disturbances to the normal healthy operation of the eye
Certain environmental conditions
Aging
Various diseases and disorders.

## BEHAVIORAL DISTURBANCES

Among the most common causes of dry eye are disturbances that disrupt the blink process or numb the surface of the eye. These disturbances in turn interfere with the production and distribution of tears. They are "behavioral" in nature; in other words, they result from activities we choose to do, such as spending long hours in front of a computer or wearing contact lenses.

One common way healthy blinking can be disrupted is by the simple act of concentration—staring or gazing at a particular object, be it a computer screen, a long highway, or a good book—for long periods. We tend to blink less frequently when we focus in this way, because the brain in effect overrides the involuntary blink mechanism to allow maximum concentration. When our blink rate slows down, evaporation on the surface of the eye speeds up, and symptoms of dry eye can appear.

### Computer Use and Other Close Activities

Over the past twenty years, computers have become almost as necessary to our everyday lives as telephones. Many jobs require sitting in front of a computer for much of the workday, and even if the computer is not needed for the job, it is frequently used at home for an infinite range of activities from paying bills to researching a vacation to playing games. Consequently, many of us habitually spend long hours in front of the computer screen, which has led to high degrees of eyestrain, eye fatigue, burning, irritation, redness, blurred vision, and excessively dry eyes, a problem experts have begun calling computer vision syndrome (see Chapter 11).

Computers are not the only culprits. Prolonged television viewing and reading can also cause reduced blink rate. Even other close work such as sewing, knitting, needlework, or other crafts can have a similar effect. And do not forget that the use of portable handheld gadgets such as PDAs, cell phones, game devices, and iPods can also cause symptoms.

The solution is relatively simple: Remind yourself to blink purposefully every few minutes as you work at a computer screen, watch television, read, or work at any activity where you find yourself focusing intently for long periods. Also, before you start any work that involves close, intense visual activity, place an artificial tear in each eye and repeat every hour.

## Driving

Driving, particularly extensive long-distance driving, also demands intense focusing, which can result in a low or reduced blink rate, which in turn can lead to symptoms of dry eye. Long-distance driving can further exacerbate dry eye when the driver (or the passengers) is exposed to turbulent air currents from either the air-conditioning or the heating system, and especially when riding in a convertible.

As you are driving, remind yourself to blink regularly, and use artificial tears every hour or so. Avoid riding in convertibles unless you wear moisture chamber glasses (see Chapter 10). Redirect the louvers of the car's air-conditioning or heating units away from your face, and use a low fan speed. It is helpful, especially in sunny or bright weather, to wear sunglasses while driving. Stop every few hours to get out of the vehicle, stretch, and "wake up" by splashing some cold water on your face (see Chapter 11).

### Sports

Certain sports can leave the surface of the eyes vulnerable to tear film disruptions. Bicycling, sailing, or skating (ice or in-line), for example, leaves the eyes exposed to strong air currents that increase tear evaporation and cause mild to extreme dry eye. Downhill skiing can pose particular problems: not only are the eyes subject to strong air currents, but they are often exposed to frigid temperatures, high altitudes, and dry air.

To cope with sports-related dry eye problems, optimize tear film with artificial tear supplements, and use moisture chamber glasses or goggles with an ultraviolet blocker designed for your sport (see Chapter 11).

### Contact Lens Wear

Dry eye is a common problem among contact lens wearers; indeed, dry eye is their most common complaint. Although today's soft lenses are less likely to nick the conjunctiva or cornea the way the old-fashioned hard lenses often did, soft lenses tend to absorb tear film, potentially causing erosion of the cornea and conjunctiva, as well as causing an allergic response called giant papillary conjunctivitis (GPC). In addition, long-term contact lens wear tends to decrease nerve sensation on the surface of the cornea, which in turn affects the stimulation of new tears as well as the blink rate. If the situation is allowed to persist over time, the result, of course, is dry eye. (See Chapter 7 for an in-depth discussion.)

## ENVIRONMENTAL CONDITIONS

Another common cause of dry eye syndrome is the climate and the state of the environment. Here I mean not only the vast outdoors in the region where you reside, but the microclimates of your home, office, automobile, and any other place where you spend extended periods.

## Indoor and Outdoor Climates

Hot, dry, and windy climates, especially those at high altitudes, frequently cause or exacerbate dry eye syndrome. These environmental conditions tend to increase tear evaporation in some people. Years of chronic exposure to bright sunlight can lead to meibomian gland dysfunction with evaporative dry eye. The ultraviolet rays can also lead to degeneration of the ocular surface tissues, which in turn can affect tear stimulation and distribution. Air pollution is yet another cause.

Indoor climates, either at home or at work, can be problematic in terms of dry eye. For example, central heating or air conditioning can cause dry eye, especially direct exposure to blasts of warm or cool air from heaters, air conditioners (especially high-velocity air-conditioner fans), and ceiling louvers distributing cool air. Even ceiling fans are a problem, especially in warm climates where many people position huge ceiling fans in the rooms they use most often, especially family rooms, living rooms, and bedrooms (often directly over the bed, which should be avoided).

Dry eye sufferers need to anticipate problems and be aware of their environment. They should avoid sitting near heating or cooling vents, especially in a situation where they sit or work for several hours each day. People suffering from advanced cases of dry eye also need to beware of sitting near air-conditioning or heating units in restaurants, theaters, airplanes, or other public places.

At home one can take control of the environment more easily. For example, it is helpful to install humidifiers in various rooms. You might want to invest in a gadget called a hygrometer, which measures moisture content in the air; you could then ensure that the air is sufficiently moist to ease dry eye, but not so humid as to advance the development of mold. Another personal solution is moisture chamber glasses, which are quite fashionable these days. For more home remedies, see Chapter 11.

### Smoking

Cigarette smoke, whether from your own cigarettes or from secondhand smoke, can cause or exacerbate dry eye. (Cigar and pipe smoke are equally troublesome.) In recent years, owing to more stringent laws in some cities and the high cost of cigarettes, smoking has decreased to some extent. Yet it remains an extremely serious health problem. We all know that smoking is responsible for a high rate of death by heart disease, emphysema, stroke, lung, and other types of cancer. However, smoking is also known to increase risk for age-related macular degeneration, cataracts, and—not surprisingly—dry eye.

Frankly, the best remedy for smoking-related dry eye (or any other smoking-related health problem) is to stop or limit smoking. If the problem is secondhand smoke, insist that smokers in your home or office smoke outside. Avoid places where smoking is permitted, such as bars or restaurants. If you must be around smoke for some reason, irrigate your eyes with sterile saline a few times during the day to rid your tear film of toxic particles.

## AGING

Aging is commonly considered a cause of dry eye syndrome, but of course it is not simply growing older that brings on the dry eye symptoms. It is the fact that many diseases (such as Parkinson's), disorders (glaucoma, cataracts), and other health problems (especially hormone abnormalities related to menopause) usually associated with older people are closely related to dry eye syndrome. The relationship between aging and dry eye syndrome is complicated and multifaceted and is covered in detail in Chapter 5.

## VARIOUS DISEASES AND DISORDERS

Dry eye syndrome is closely related to a host of diseases and disorders. In some cases, the disease in question directly damages the tear glands, causing some form of dry eye, either aqueous tear deficient dry eye or evaporative dry eye. In other cases, mild to severe dry eye may develop secondarily as a symptom of the disease. Most cases of dry eye are related to localized eye disorders; however, some of the most severe cases are associated with systemic diseases.

## Localized Eye Disorders

In many cases, dry eye can develop because of diseases, disorders, and other health problems that affect the eyes specifically. Among these is primary acquired lacrimal gland disease (also known as non-Sjögren's aqueous tear deficiency), one of the two most common causes of dry eye. The other is meibomian gland dysfunction. Other localized eye problems associated with dry eye include anterior blepharitis, allergies, lagophthalmos (incomplete eye closure), secondary blepharospasm, stroke, delayed tear clearance, conjunctivochalasis, ocular herpes, anterior basement membrane dystrophy (a disorder involving the irregular surface of the cornea), and eye surgeries such as LASIK. Less common causes include radiation therapy around the eye and acute emergencies such as chemical or thermal burns to the eye.

### Primary Acquired Lacrimal Gland Disease

Primary acquired lacrimal gland disease is possibly the most common cause of dry eye syndrome; one might even say it *is* dry eye syndrome. It involves a breakdown of the functioning of the lacrimal glands; in other words, the lacrimal glands fail to secrete sufficient aqueous tears, and the classic dry eye symptoms appear (red irritated eyes, dryness, and vision fluctuation). Primary lacrimal gland disease is usually age related, which basically means that the tear glands have grown older and are just not functioning as well as they once did. Some research indicates that primary lacrimal gland disease may also be caused by reduction of the level of androgens (hormones) in the system, making it more a systemic problem than a localized one. For more information about primary acquired lacrimal gland disease, see Chapter 5.

### Meibomian Gland Dysfunction

Meibomian gland dysfunction (also referred to as MGD, meibomitis, and posterior blepharitis) is also a leading cause of dry eye syndrome. It is a very complicated disease, but typically involves inflammation of the meibomian, or lipid secreting, glands in the eyelids caused by a blockage of the gland orifice at the lid margin. The blockage may be caused by swelling due to allergies or from anterior blepharitis. Meibomian gland dysfunction may relate to hormonal changes, as well as to dietary habits that affect the thickness and viscosity of the meibum. The result sometimes is cheese-like gland secretions or, in other cases, a hard wax plug at the gland orifice that ends up clogging the gland. Another type of meibomian gland dysfunction, seborrheic lid disease, features excessive lipid secretion (although the glands do not become obstructed) that causes irritation to the eyes. The bottom line is that the meibomian glands produce too much oil, too little oil, or oil that is too thick or otherwise of abnormal quality. As a result, the tear film becomes unstable, evaporates too quickly from the surface of the eye, and ultimately develops into evaporative dry eye.

Treating meibomian gland dysfunction and evaporative dry eye is a complicated process and may involve physical, medicinal, nutritional, and hormonal therapies. These are discussed in detail in Chapter 10.

### Anterior Blepharitis

Blepharitis is a general term typically used to mean inflammation of the eyelid margin involving redness and irritation. Anterior blepharitis usually refers specifically to a bacterial infection of the lash follicles, with crusting or flaking around the lash root, as opposed to posterior blepharitis, which involves the meibomian glands and meibomian gland dysfunction. Although anterior blepharitis does not directly cause dry eye, inflammation of the eyelid margin and the lash follicles can quickly lead to posterior blepharitis, meibomian gland dysfunction, and evaporative dry eye.

### Allergies, Toxicities, and Sensitivities

Allergies—and sometimes even the treatments for allergies—are common causes of dry eye. Inflammation of the conjunctiva can result from an allergic response to dust, mold, mildew, animal dander, dirty air, and many other substances. If it becomes chronic, this inflammation of the ocular surface numbs the eye and short-circuits the message to the lacrimal glands to produce tears. The inflammation also destabilizes the tear film and can cause evaporative dry eye.

Ironically and unfortunately, eyedrops designed to treat allergic eyes can worsen the pain of existing dry eye. Further, drops meant to treat dry eye may contain preservatives that can cause a toxic or inflammatory eye reaction or, less commonly, an allergic reaction.

If you suffer from allergies as well as dry eye, be sure your eye doctor is fully aware of your allergic problems. Chapter 6 presents a fuller discussion of allergies and dry eye.

### Problems with Lid Closure

When the eyelids do not close properly or completely, the surface of the eye is left exposed and dry eye can develop. Many diseases and disorders involve problems with lid closure; here are a few of the more common problems.

Lagophthalmos is a condition in which the eyelids do not close completely; nocturnal lagophthalmos is when this occurs during sleep. As a result, the exposed eye can become excessively dry, and dry eye symptoms can develop.

Bell's palsy is an abnormality of the facial nerves that manifests as a weakness or paralysis of the muscles on one side of the face. Since paralyzed facial muscles often impede the blinking process as well as prevent the eye from closing completely, a bout with Bell's palsy can bring on dry eye.

Lid ectropion and lid laxity are usually age-related conditions where typically the lower lid does not properly hug or cover the eyeball. With ectropion, the lid rolls outward away from the eye, creating a large space where tears may well up and not be distributed properly across the ocular surface. The welled-up tears may overflow, causing a problem with excessive tears even though the eye is dry. With lid laxity, although the lower lid does not roll away from the eye, it is loose and may droop; the exposed ocular surface area increases and may then become dry.

Congenital ptosis, sometimes called droopy eyelid, results from a weakness in the muscle of the eyelid or interference in the nerve supply to the eyelid muscle. (Adults may also develop ptosis as a result of certain diseases, disorders, or injury.) If a child is born with drooping eyelids hanging over the pupil, surgery may be necessary to raise the lid in order to avoid impaired vision. Because of the abnormal lid muscles, these children may be unable to close the lid effectively, promoting severe dry eye.

Cosmetic surgery in adults with droopy eyelids (ptosis surgery), baggy lids (blepharoplasty), or a full facelift, if not properly done, can cause problems such as incomplete lid closure with exposure (lagophthalmos) or abnormal tear flow and distribution from altered lid movements, which in turn can lead to dry eye.

### Secondary Blepharospasm or Eyelid Spasm

Irritation from dry eye may lead to eyelid spasm, or frequent blinking. Persistent eyelid spasm may cause increased irritation, resulting in a cycle of more forceful spasms. *Secondary blepharospasm* is different from *essential blepharospasm,* in which the forceful spasms are the result of a neurologic disorder.

BOX 7

**Case Study: Claudia**

A 50-year-old compassionate, dedicated nurse who became very upset with her gradually failing vision, Claudia was born with congenital ptosis. She had her eyelids lifted appropriately at about 2 years of age, so that she could learn to see. Because of her abnormal lids, she could not close them completely, leaving her cornea exposed and dry. Over the years she developed corneal scarring from recurrent corneal infections and excessive dryness. The cumulative effect was that she was no longer readily able to do "fine" work, including reading the small print on medications and syringes. Her dry eye was starting to make it impossible for her to do her job.

When I evaluated her, I found that she had inadequate tear production, and that some of her few precious tears were being distributed to the outer corner of her eye rather than across her eye, owing to a severe case of conjunctivochalasis (a pleating of the conjunctiva). I carefully removed the corneal scars, performed a punctal occlusion to increase her tear volume, and reconstructed the ocular surface using amnionic membrane to smooth the surface pleats and minimize risk of recurrent scarring of the cornea.

Claudia has been back at work for almost a year. She can read the 20/20 line on the eye chart and says "this is the best vision I have ever had."

HAVE YOU SEEN?

**Courtesy of Claudia Jenkins**

Dedicated to
My parents, who gave me sight,
and to
Dr. Maskin, who restored it

Have you seen today?
I have.
How bright and sharp the world is.
Raindrops are crystal clear, distinct, and individual.
The color green, so many shades; look there, how that bird can sing.

Have you seen today?
I have.

My, my hair is so very gray. But do I care?
The colors I see no longer muted, pale, or the same.

Have you seen today?
I have.

The words jumping off a page, no longer trying to see what I know is there.
How clear, how sharp the day really is.

Have you seen today?
I have.

And oh my, I can't wait to see tomorrow.

Have you seen today?

### Stroke

In stroke, the blood flow to the brain is disrupted and brain cells are damaged or die from lack of oxygen. Many symptoms can occur, including loss of sensation in an arm, leg, or along one side of the body; dizziness; slurred speech; difficulty thinking clearly or speaking; imbalance and falling; and fainting. A stroke can also present serious eye problems, including partial loss of vision, double vision, and if facial muscles are affected, an inability to blink that can evolve into dry eye. Also, stroke can lead to loss of sensation in the corneal nerves, which cuts off the message to the tear glands to secrete and to the lids to blink. The outcome again can be dry eye.

### Delayed Tear Clearance

Sometimes the tear duct that leads to the nose can become partially blocked as a result of aged lax tissues or swollen allergic tissues, leading to a situation known as delayed tear clearance. When the tears are not permitted to drain, "dirty" tears containing allergens, toxins, and other irritants accumulate on the surface of the eye. The eye may then become chronically inflamed, which in turn numbs its surface and inhibits the message to the lacrimal glands to secrete fresh tears; dry eye develops.

When the tear clearance drainage system is blocked owing to infection, the surrounding tissues that form at the inner angle of the eye (the canthus) become swollen, red, and tender. Treatment with antibiotics is required and in some cases a new tear duct needs to be created. If the site of infection is the tear drain sac in the nose, the condition is called dacryocystitis.

### Conjunctivochalasis

This common disorder can result from overexposure to the sun's ultraviolet rays or chronic surface inflammation, among other reasons. With conjunctivochalasis, the conjunctiva loses its elasticity, becomes wrinkled or pleated, and ends up drooping over the lid margin. Because it is "loose," the wrinkled or pleated conjunctiva may be squeezed between the lid and eyeball resulting in a painful pinched feeling. Blinking, especially hard blinking, simply makes the problem worse. Also, the abnormal tissue alters the tear flow and distribution, thereby causing dry eye symptoms.

### Ocular Herpes

Herpes keratitis, or ocular herpes, is a type of corneal infection usually brought on by the Type I herpes simplex virus, the same virus responsible for cold sores on the lips. (It can also be brought on by Type II herpes simplex, which causes genital herpes, or by herpes zoster, which is responsible for shingles.) The symptoms including blurred vision, strong sensitivity to light, redness, and disruption of the blink reflex. During the first outbreak, the eye experiences pain and waters excessively, but ultimately the sensation in the cornea is reduced and dry eye may set in. Ocular herpes almost always affects just one eye, but in rare cases can affect both. In addition, like other herpetic infections, it can be controlled but not cured and may often recur.

### Anterior Basement Membrane Dystrophy and Recurrent Erosion Syndrome

Anterior basement membrane dystrophy (also called map-dot-fingerprint dystrophy) is a common defect that results in an irregular corneal surface and, in some situations, can lead to dry eye symptoms when the overlying tear film becomes unstable. It is primarily an inherited defect that affects the thin layer of connective tissue at the base of the deepest cornea epithelial cell level, but it can occur as an abnormal healing response if the epithelium is nicked with a fingernail or a mascara brush, for example. This abnormal layer of connective tissue leads to a reduction in the adherence of the overlying epithelial cells. Although most patients experience only fluctuating vision without discomfort, some patients develop blurred vision and exquisitely painful recurrent epithelial erosions (recurrent erosion syndrome). The erosions typically develop when the sufferer wakes up in the morning and the eyelid pulls a layer of epithelial "skin" off the cornea. This syndrome is referred to as recurrent because it may be difficult to heal and recurs repeatedly.

## LASIK and Other Surgeries

Vision-corrective surgeries numb the nerves on the surface of the eye and interrupt messages to the tear glands and the blink mechanism. They can—and frequently do—result in dry eye. LASIK (or laser in situ keratomileusis) is a common refractive procedure to correct nearsightedness, farsightedness, and astigmatism. With LASIK (and other similar refractive surgeries) the nerve endings in the cornea are cut or ablated during the procedure. The nerves, now numb, are at least transiently unable to effectively direct the tear glands to produce tears or the eyelids to blink. Dry eye syndrome is a frequent consequence.

Corneal and other surface ocular sensation can also be disrupted by cataract operations, corneal transplants, retinal detachment repair, and other ocular surgical procedures, with dry eye again being a possible consequence.

## Radiation Treatment

Radiation is a common local treatment for various cancers and is sometimes used for other diseases. With the correct dosage of radiation, normal cells suffer little or no damage; however, radiation treatment may produce side effects, including fatigue, nausea, vomiting, and hair loss. Dry eye can develop after radiation, especially when it is used to treat cancers of the eye or face, and if the eye is not adequately shielded. In this situation, the radiation damages the tear glands or causes a scarring reaction that obstructs the glands so that they cannot discharge their secretions.

### Chemical and Thermal Burns

Chemical or thermal burns to the eye resulting from accidental exposure to extreme temperatures or from a toxic substance, such as lye or bleach, touching the surface of the eye may have a severe effect on the tear glands' ability to function. Although dry eye may result, these cases are typically catastrophic. They often lead to blindness and require heroic efforts to save the eye and restore sight over time.

## Systemic Diseases

Individuals with dry eye syndrome may also suffer from a serious systemic illness, such as Sjögren's syndrome, rheumatoid arthritis, lupus, or diabetes, that turns out to be related to their chronically dry eyes.

### Sjögren's Syndrome and Related Diseases

Sjögren's syndrome, a frequent cause of aqueous tear deficient dry eye, has come to be considered the benchmark for serious dry eye. Not all people who suffer from dry eye have Sjögren's syndrome—not by a long shot. In fact, not all cases of aqueous tear deficient dry eye are related to Sjögren's. However, because of the nature and severity of the disease, and because other serious diseases are often associated with Sjögren's syndrome, it is important to review Sjögren's and a few other systemic diseases commonly associated with dry eye.

#### *Sjögren's Syndrome*

Sjögren's syndrome is a chronic autoimmune disease in which the body's immune system mistakenly attacks its own moisture-producing glands, including the saliva glands and the tear glands. General fatigue, dry mouth, and dry eye are typical symptoms. Sjögren's can also affect other organs, such as the kidneys, lungs, liver, gastrointestinal tract, and peripheral or central nervous system. Two to three million Americans suffer from Sjögren's syndrome. While it can affect men and younger people, as many as 90 percent of sufferers are women, and most of those are middle-aged, postmenopausal women.

Aqueous tear deficient dry eye is the most characteristic feature of Sjögren's syndrome. The disease destroys the tear-producing cells of the lacrimal gland, and dry eye develops because the supply of aqueous tears is largely and chronically reduced. (Inadequate mucin and meibomian gland dysfunction may also play a role.) Sjögren's syndrome tends to show up with certain other autoimmune disorders such as rheumatoid arthritis and lupus erythematosus.

Although at the moment there is no cure for Sjögren's syndrome, mild dry eye related to Sjögren's syndrome can initially be managed with artificial tears. If it is not treated adequately, Sjögren's syndrome may lead to serious dry eye as well as infection, ulceration, and perforation of the cornea, visual loss, and blindness.

### *Rheumatoid Arthritis*

Rheumatoid arthritis is a disorder that affects the joints of the fingers, wrists, toes, or other joints in the body, which become painful, swollen, stiff, and possibly deformed. In severe cases, inflammation may affect the covering of the heart and the lungs, as well as nerves and blood vessels. Rheumatoid arthritis is an autoimmune disorder, meaning that the body attacks its own tissues. The disorder usually starts in early adulthood but can develop at any age, and it affects women three times more frequently than men. When associated with Sjögren's syndrome, the lacrimal glands and salivary glands are also affected, making both the eyes and the mouth dry.

### *Systemic Lupus Erythematosus*

Lupus erythematosus, or lupus, as it is commonly known, is another autoimmune disorder in which the body's immune system attacks tissues and organ systems throughout the body as though they were foreign, causing widespread inflammation. Organs such as heart, lung, and kidney may be involved in addition to muscles, joints, and blood cells. The skin may be involved; lupus frequently features a red, blotchy, butterfly-shaped rash over the cheeks and bridge of the nose. The disease affects nine times as many women as men, usually those of childbearing age. As in rheumatoid arthritis associated with Sjögren's syndrome, the lacrimal glands and salivary glands come under attack, leading to dry eye and dry mouth.

## Non-Sjögren's-Related Tear Deficiencies

Many systemic diseases and disorders, aside from those related to Sjögren's syndrome, feature a characteristic aqueous tear deficiency.

### *Secondary Lacrimal Gland Diseases*

Secondary lacrimal gland diseases are systemic disorders that can destroy lacrimal gland tissue, thus inhibiting tear production and secretion. Examples are sarcoidosis (a disease of unknown origin marked by the formation of lesions or tumors that appear especially in the liver, lungs, skin, and lymph nodes), graft-versus-host disease (a type of incompatibility reaction of transplanted bone marrow cells against the host tissues), and HIV-AIDS.

### *Diabetes Mellitus*

Diabetes is a disorder in which the pancreas produces insufficient or no insulin, the hormone responsible for the transport of glucose into cells for their energy needs and into the liver and fat cells for storage. Because of insufficient insulin, the level of glucose in the blood becomes abnormally high, causing excessive urination and constant thirst and hunger; because of the body's inability to store or use glucose, weight loss and chronic fatigue develop.

Many people (as many as 14 million Americans by some studies) suffer from diabetes, 90 percent suffering Type II (non-insulin-related, adult-onset diabetes) and 10 percent suffering from Type I (insulin-dependent diabetes that typically occurs in childhood). Both types can affect vision.

Diabetes is a complex disorder, but among its most severe complications—if the diabetes is not controlled properly—are eye problems, especially retinopathy (damage to the retina, the light-sensitive area at the back of the eye) and cataracts. In more severe cases, diabetes can also cause decreased sensitivity to the cornea, which can disrupt tear production and ultimately lead to aqueous tear deficient dry eye.

### *Ocular Cicatricial Pemphigoid*

Cicatricial pemphigoid is a chronic autoimmune disease that features scarring of conjunctival and at times other mucosal tissues such as in the nose, throat, esophagus, urethra, vagina, and anus. With regard to the eyes, it appears as a chronic inflammation of the conjunctiva with scarring of the ocular surface tissues that may cause obstruction of the lacrimal gland secretory ducts and result in aqueous tear deficiency. The scarring process can also cause a dry and unstable tear film by obstruction of the meibomian gland orifices and loss of conjunctival goblet cells. This chronic but progressive disease may leave the eyelids scarred and attached to the eyeball, thereby inhibiting normal eye movement; further, the patient may become blind from cornea scarring. A similar scarring reaction may develop from chronic use of certain topical glaucoma medications, a condition called pseudopemphigoid.

### *Stevens-Johnson Syndrome*

Stevens-Johnson syndrome is an acute, life-threatening, systemic disease that causes rash, skin peeling, and sores on the mucous membranes, like an extremely severe burn. Many cases are caused by infection, while others result from a reaction to certain drugs including antibiotics, barbiturates, and anti-inflammatory drugs. Sometimes no cause can be identified. Blisters break out on the mucous membranes lining the mouth, throat, anus, genitals, and eyes.

With regard to the eyes, the lids become very painful and swell, and the eyes may become filled with a thick discharge that seals them shut, putting the corneas at risk for infection. Typically, patients are hospitalized and treated in a burn unit. After recovery, these patients have severe dry eye owing to extensive scarring of all tear glands. This catastrophic disease may dry out the normal wettable mucosal surface of the eye, leaving it scaly with loss of luster and thick folds of tissue; it frequently leads to blindness.

## Other Systemic Diseases

Most systemic diseases associated with dry eye involve the destruction of the lacrimal glands. However, other diseases attack other facets of the lacrimal functional unit, including the meibomian glands, the goblet cells, and the blink mechanism, and can result in other forms of dry eye.

### Rosacea

Rosacea (also known as acne rosacea) is a chronic skin disorder in which the cheeks and nose are abnormally red, and deep-seated pustules involve the sebaceous glands on the skin on the face (think of W. C. Fields). Rosacea can affect the meibomian glands in the eyelids, resulting in severe blepharitis, which in turn can alter the production of tear lipids and lead to evaporative dry

BOX 8

**Case Study: Homeless Man**

In our culture, we rarely see vitamin-A deficiency because despite the supposed fight against obesity, we are usually well nourished and receive sufficient vitamins, including vitamin A. However, I did have one case that I found fascinating.

A colleague called to say he had a young patient who seemed to be quickly losing his vision. The patient's corneas were severely ulcerated and becoming opaque. My friend was worried, and of course so was his patient.

The man, who was only in his thirties, walked into my office with the help of a cane. He was absolutely emaciated. I could see by the nature of the "punched-out" ulcers on his cornea that he had a vitamin-A deficiency. After ordering a blood test to confirm, I prescribed an injection of vitamin A and supplements. (Also, my office staff bought him lunch.) Within a couple of weeks his ulcers were healed. His vision soon returned, and he returned—this time without the cane.

eye. The severe blepharitis may create a highly inflamed ocular surface, which can reduce goblet cell densities in the conjunctiva and thus further destabilize the tear film.

### Vitamin-A Deficiency

Goblet cells of the conjunctiva may be damaged from a variety of systemic inflammatory diseases affecting the ocular surface, including rosacea, ocular cicatricial pemphigoid, and Stevens-Johnson syndrome. Vitamin-A deficiency (or xerophthalmia) is a well-known but rare cause of goblet cell deficiency; it is caused by malnutrition, specifically a vitamin-A deficiency. (In the United States and other industrialized countries, vitamin-A deficiency from malnutrition is very rare. When the deficiency does occur in industrialized countries, it is usually the result of intestinal and liver diseases or of digestive tract surgery.) Vitamin A is essential for normal health of the corneal epithelium, and its deficiency causes loss of goblet cells. The conjunctiva is left with a dull irregular surface that becomes scaly and nonwettable. Therefore this disease creates a severe dry eye and abnormal cornea, which leads to erosions and ulceration.

### Graves' Disease

Graves' disease (also known as thyroid eye disease or thyroid orbitopathy) is the most common cause of proptosis (protruding eye) in adults. It is an autoimmune disease that involves an overactive and enlarged thyroid gland. Bulging eyes may result, and the eyelids are typically retracted. As a result of the greater exposure of the surface of the eyes and problems with blinking, severe dry eye symptoms may develop over time.

## WHEN THE PROBLEM IS *NOT* DRY EYE SYNDROME

A number of eye diseases and disorders may "present" (to use a common medical expression) as dry eye syndrome in that the symptoms are similar. In fact, many of these problems are caused by something other than a breakdown in tear production or evaporation. Here are a few of the more common problems that may initially look like dry eye, but are not. It is useful to remember that although these disorders are not technically dry eye, they may, if inadequately treated, develop into dry eye.

### Itchy Eyes and Eyelids

Eyes and eyelids can become itchy for many reasons. A true itch, like that of a mosquito bite, suggests an allergic disorder rather

BOX 9

**Medication-Induced Causes of Dry Eye**

Many medications can cause or exacerbate dry eye. These include:

Allergy medications (particularly antihistamines)
Decongestants
Diuretics
Birth control pills
Hormone replacement therapies (HRT)
Antidepressants
Sleeping pills
Medications for heart disease and Parkinson's disease

If you have recently developed dry eye, consider whether you have just begun taking medication for some other ailment such as an allergy or a preexisting disease. If you already have dry eye syndrome, perhaps a new medication is making your eye problems worse. Check with your doctor and read up on the side effects of your medications. Perhaps your doctor can prescribe an alternative medication that will not affect you as much. (For example, a topical allergy medication or one that is locally delivered, such as a nasal spray, may be preferable to an oral, or systemic, medication. If a systemic med is needed, a liquid is preferred as it is easier to titrate.) Do not stop taking a prescribed medication if you start to experience eye pain, but do check with your primary care physician—and your eye doctor—as soon as possible.

BOX 10

**Crazy Lashes**

One of the most common causes of the sensation of a foreign object in the eye is an aberrant growth of the eyelashes, a problem called trichiasis. The eyelashes grow inward, toward the eye, instead of outward. (A related problem, called distichaisis, is characterized by two or more rows of lashes.) The lashes can actually impale the cornea, causing annoying pain and damaging the cornea's surface. Ulceration is possible. Trichiasis can be treated by removal of the lashes, but often they grow back. Permanent treatment involves destruction of the follicles of the eyelashes, first trying electrolysis, freezing, or radiosurgical techniques before attempting surgical removal.

than tear deficiency. It is true that allergies often accompany dry eye and can even cause evaporative and aqueous tear deficient dry eye. But usually a true simple itch without other symptoms has nothing to do with dry eye.

## Foreign Objects

Sometimes if we get "something in our eye," like a loose eyelash; some sand or dirt; a fragment of metal, plastic, or wood; or any other actual foreign particle, our eyes will tear up, turn red, and possibly hurt tremendously—all of which could be symptoms of dry eye. However, with dry eye, the sensation of a foreign body is usually the result of a sensitive corneal nerve, which became sensitive because of problematic tear production or evaporation. In other words, with dry eye no actual foreign body exists; it just feels that way.

### Referred Eye Pain

Although eye pain is a common symptom of dry eye, not all eye pain indicates dry eye syndrome. I have even diagnosed patients who thought they had eye pain and had nothing at all wrong with their eyes! The pain is real, but it is referred pain (the most common form of which is known as occipital neuralgia)—which means that it was generated by another part of the body, such as the back of the neck, but sent the message to the brain that the eyes hurt. In order to find the true source of referred eye pain, your doctor needs to examine your head and neck. Often referred pain can be effectively diagnosed with an injection of lidocaine, a common local anesthetic. Treatment may include massage and heat applications.

### Sties, Chalazions, Tumors, and Other Lid Masses

Sties, chalazions, plugged oil glands, and other swellings or masses on the eyelid may become inflamed, causing pain and redness and decreased vision with foreign body sensation. All can simulate dry eye, but are separate disorders that require separate treatments.

### Floppy Eyelid Syndrome

Floppy eyelid syndrome is characterized by lax or flaccid upper eyelids that "flop" into an abnormal inverted position during sleep. It most frequently develops in overweight, middle-aged males, although occasionally it is seen in women. Since the eyelids are inverted, the conjunctiva lining the upper lid rubs against the pillowcase. Like dry eye, symptoms (which may show up in both eyes, but usually only in one if you sleep on one side) include general eye irritation and redness due to an inflamed upper lid, itching, and a stringy mucus discharge, particularly immediately after waking up. Patients may also suffer from sleep apnea.

## Entropion and Lid Imbrication

Entropion and lid imbrication are eyelid problems characterized by the turning inward of the eyelids (entropion) so that lashes can abrade the cornea or the improper relationship or overlapping of the upper and lower lids (imbrication). Symptoms include excess tears, foreign body sensation, redness, and fluctuating vision, all of which may inaccurately suggest dry eye. Lid surgery may be needed.

## Corneal Problems

A number of disorders that affect the cornea look like dry eye, and may even lead to dry eye, but are not dry eye. Other corneal disorders may develop because of the presence of dry eye. Here are a few examples.

A pterygium is a thickening of the conjunctiva that extends across the margin of the cornea toward the center of the eye. It is caused by prolonged exposure to hot, dusty, and dry environments with bright sunlight, and occurs frequently in tropical areas. Closely related to pterygium is a pinguecula, a benign degenerative growth at the junction of the cornea and the conjunctiva, which can become inflamed and irritated. Pingueculae (they are usually plural) may also be caused by overexposure to ultraviolet light; they occur most frequently among people who spend a great deal of time outdoors in strong sunlight. Both pinguecula and pterygium may cause redness in the eyes, irritation, and blurry vision, all symptoms of dry eye disease. Furthermore, these lesions can be stimulated and exacerbated by dry eye syndrome. In other words, they do not cause dry eye, but dry eye may cause them.

Dry eye may also lead to superior limbic keratoconjunctivitis and filamentary keratitis. Superior limbic keratoconjunctivitis (SLK) is inflammation and redness on the top part of the eyeball at the junction of the colored and white parts, while filamentary keratitis presents with mucus filaments attached to the cornea. These problems may have symptoms similar to dry eye, including redness, foreign body sensation, pain, and fluctuating vision; they do not cause dry eye syndrome, although they can be induced or exacerbated by dry eye. Thygeson's keratitis, which features a foreign body sensation and fluctuating vision similar to dry eye, is completely unrelated.

## THE CHICKEN, THE EGG, AND DRY EYE SYNDROME

You have probably begun to realize that dry eye syndrome is often characterized by the proverbial "chicken and egg" situation. In other words, which condition came first, the dry eyes or the related eye problem? And if it's dry eye, which type is it—aqueous tear deficient or evaporative? Can one type lead to the other?

Blepharitis (both anterior and posterior) is a perfect example. You can have a relatively benign case of anterior blepharitis in which the lash follicles are infected and cause swelling of the lid margin. This then quickly leads to posterior blepharitis, because the meibomian glands become obstructed and evaporative dry eye develops. Conversely, you may have a full-blown case of posterior blepharitis or meibomian gland dysfunction, which promotes increased bacteria on the lid, or anterior blepharitis.

Allergies and sensitivities versus aqueous tear deficiency pose another type of chicken-and-egg situation. You can have an allergic reaction resulting in chronic inflammation of the surface of the eye, which can also numb the surface of the eye. The message to the lacrimal glands shuts down, insufficient tears are produced, and the surface of the eye becomes further inflamed. A vicious cycle evolves, which may end up as aqueous tear deficient dry eye. On the other hand, the aqueous tear deficiency may have occurred first. Without enough tears to wash it away, an offending toxin or allergen gains increased contact time on the eye. Also, without adequate tears, anything that gets into the eye is inadequately diluted, creating a potential toxic concentration.

Aqueous tear deficiency versus meibomian gland dysfunction is yet another example. Surface inflammation from aqueous tear deficiency causes inflammation of the lid margin and obstruction of the gland orifice; obstruction of the gland orifice leads to meibomian gland dysfunction and tear instability, and evaporative dry eye results. Conversely, meibomian gland dysfunction is associated with chronic surface inflammation, which leads to reduced sensation on the ocular surface, which leads to aqueous tear deficiency.

## There Goes the Neighborhood

Closely related to the chicken-and-egg situation is the concept of "there goes the neighborhood." Once dry eye—aqueous tear deficient or evaporative—develops, a number of other diseases and disorders may show up. For example, dry eye can cause or exacerbate (and often accompanies) diseases and disorders such as recurrent erosion syndrome, pterygium, pingueculae, SLK, filamentary keratitis, and anterior blepharitis.

Obviously, the causes—and the effects—of dry eye syndrome are complex and multifaceted. A few require an even closer look because they are so common and affect so many people. We turn in the next chapters to aging, allergies, contact-lens-related dry eye, and refractive surgery.

CHAPTER

# 5

# Aging and Gender

Myth

*Tear glands wear out as we age for no apparent reason—simply because we are older.*

Fact

*Increasing evidence indicates that hormone deficiencies that occur as we age may lead to dry eye.*

Viewed from a certain perspective, it might be said that aging is the most common cause of dry eye syndrome. However, it is not just the reality of growing older that brings on dry eye symptoms. It is also the fact that many diseases (such as rheumatoid arthritis), disorders (blepharitis), and other health problems (especially hormone changes related to menopause) usually associated with aging are closely related to dry eye.

Among the diseases, primary acquired lacrimal gland disease (also known as non-Sjögren's aqueous tear deficiency) is the most common cause of dry eye syndrome. Primary acquired lacrimal gland disease involves the breakdown of the functioning of the lacrimal glands; in other words, the lacrimal glands fail to produce sufficient aqueous tears, and the classic dry eye symptoms appear (a gritty or scratchy feeling in the eyes, red irritated eyes, excess tearing, and vision fluctuation). Primary acquired lacrimal gland disease is, indeed, almost always age related, which basically means that as the tear glands grow older, they are just not working as well as they once did. However, that is only part of the story—to use an old cliché, it is only the tip of the iceberg.

The much larger element of this "iceberg" is how we define the concept of aging. What exactly is aging? Because we tend to live longer and healthier lives these days, we've changed our definition of elderly. Not long ago, age 65 seemed old; now that perception is reserved for someone who may be 75 or 80.

From a medical or scientific point of view, one definition of aging has to do with the slow (or perhaps not so slow) decline in hormone production, especially production of the sex hormones (androgens and estrogens), in the human body. The reduction and change of human sex hormones is an extremely complex process, more so in women than in men, in that it affects women earlier in life and more profoundly. From a medical perspective, women are said to be aging when they begin perimenopause, which usually happens after age 40, but sometimes earlier. And when women experience perimenopause, they often show symptoms of dry eye. To put it differently, reduction in sex hormones appears to relate directly to dry eye.

## WOMEN, HORMONES, AND DRY EYE

One of the most compelling aspects of dry eye syndrome is that it occurs predominantly among women. Some experts have gone so far as to state that being a female is a risk factor for dry eye! Most of the women who suffer from dry eye are menopausal. In addition, a large number of women with premature ovarian failure (that is, they have gone through menopause before age 40), women who are pregnant or lactating, and women who are taking birth control pills suffer from dry eye.

At first glance, it would appear that dry eye has something to do with the so-called female hormones. Here people immediately think of estrogen; but estrogen does not appear to be the primary problem with regard to dry eye. Ironically, the opposite is true. The culprit seems to be the androgen hormones, a group of steroids that includes the male hormone testosterone.

## The Key to Dry Eye in Women

Androgen hormones are steroids that control the masculine characteristics, such as facial and body hair (including male baldness), the growth of the penis, the development of bulky muscles, and the deepening of the voice. Androgens are thought to promote aggression, a characteristically male trait. They also stimulate the secretion of sebum, which, if excessive, may cause acne, especially in teenage boys. If produced in excess in women, androgens cause the development of similar masculine features, such as increase in body hair, lowering of the voice, enlargement of the clitoris, and absence of menstruation.

Androgens are produced by specialized cells in the testes in males and in the adrenal glands in both sexes. In women, the ovaries also secrete small quantities of androgens until menopause, whereupon the production of androgens by the ovaries completely shuts down. Men, of course, generate larger quantities of androgen hormones, with more of them produced by the testes than by the adrenal glands. In men the androgen levels diminish gradually over decades, rather than relatively quickly as they do in women.

Androgens support various types of glandular tissue (most particularly the sex glands) and, as it turns out, have a significant influence on the tear glands. Since with menopause the androgen level in most women is reduced dramatically, some researchers suggest that the reduced androgen levels lead to dry eye, specifically non-Sjögren's aqueous tear-deficient dry eye due to lacrimal gland deficiency. (Because androgens also have anti-inflammatory properties, lack of androgen may lead to inflammation of the ocular surface tissues.) Some experts even believe that non-Sjögren's aqueous tear deficiency is gender specific and may not occur in males at all.

In comparison, a significantly lower than normal level of androgens is found in people suffering from Sjögren's syndrome, an autoimmune disease that is one of the primary causes of dry eye syndrome. Studies have shown that the low levels of androgens in patients suffering from Sjögren's syndrome are a major factor for the lacrimal gland dysfunction, decreased tear secretion, and consequent dry eye encountered in those patients. Perhaps not surprisingly, 90 percent of Sjögren's syndrome sufferers are women.

Finally, some studies have shown that androgens also target the meibomian glands and may regulate lipid production within this tissue, promoting the formation of the tear film's lipid layer. If androgens are reduced or deficient, meibomian gland dysfunction and evaporative dry eye may result. In rare cases, a syndrome called complete androgen insensitivity syndrome (CAIS) may occur; a mutation occurs in the androgen receptor gene, making the body unable to respond to the androgen hormone. The result, again, may be meibomian gland dysfunction and evaporative dry eye.

### Hormone Therapies for Dry Eye

It might seem obvious that a simple way to treat dry eye caused by androgen deficiency would be simply to offer some sort of hormonal treatment. Although research is still being done in this area, current investigations suggest that hormone therapy might be effective either as an eyedrop placed directly onto the surface of the eye or as a hormonal cream rubbed into the skin around the eye, including on the lid. In either case, the patient would have to be monitored for adverse effects elsewhere in the body (including the heart and liver as well as the prostate for men).

### An Exacerbating Factor

Although estrogen is not the main culprit with regard to women and dry eye, it cannot be dismissed completely. Estrogen hormones (estrogens, like androgens, are actually a group of hormones) are essential for normal female sexual development and for a healthy functioning of the female reproductive system. In women, they are produced mainly by the ovaries but are also formed in the placenta during pregnancy and in the adrenal glands. (Men produce estrogen too, but in very small amounts.)

The nature of estrogen's influence on the lacrimal gland is complex and controversial. Some researchers have found that estrogens play an important role in the anatomy and physiology of the lacrimal glands and that estrogen deficiency is related to postmenopausal dry eye. However, other researchers report that it is the presence of estrogen—as opposed to its absence—that has a negative influence on the lacrimal glands, resulting in reduced tear secretion.

Indeed, dry eye is prevalent not only among postmenopausal women (whose estrogen levels are reduced), but also among women who are pregnant, lactating, or taking estrogen supplements such as birth control pills, thus increasing the estrogen levels. Some studies have indicated that postmenopausal women who use hormone replacement therapy (HRT) have a higher prevalence of dry eye syndrome than women who have not used HRT. Those women who took estrogen alone with HRT had significantly higher rates of dry eye than those who took estrogen plus progesterone and/or progestin. Other tests have shown that estrogens may promote evaporative dry eye by antagonizing the normal meibomian gland function.

To sum up: The general conclusion is that a reduction in androgens is the primary problem with regard to dry eye and aging. It is primarily the decline in androgen levels—not the change in estrogen levels—that occurs during menopause, pregnancy, lactation, and use of estrogen-containing oral contraceptives that may lead to the development of primary acquired lacrimal gland deficiency. In women with Sjögren's syndrome, which itself is a predominantly female disease, the androgen deficiency clearly plays a significant role in both aqueous tear deficient and evaporative dry eye.

Even though estrogen is not the primary problem, it may

play a role in exacerbating dry eye syndrome. The precise role of estrogen with regard to the lacrimal gland and meibomian gland function is still uncertain, and far more research is required before these issues will be clarified.

## MEN, AGING, AND DRY EYE

Although the numbers of those affected are not nearly so great as those of affected women, men are not immune to dry eye. They do suffer from dry eye more and more as they age, but the disease tends to show up later in life than it does with women, primarily because men don't go through as dramatic a hormonal reduction process as women do.

Since research indicates that evaporative dry eye may develop as a result of androgen deficiency and androgen reduction is slower in men, it may take decades for a significant reduction to have an effect in men with regard to dry eye. The exception seems to be when antiandrogen therapy is used to treat prostate cancer; studies have shown that meibomian gland dysfunction and evaporative dry eye may develop in these cases.

## GERIATRIC ILLNESSES

The challenges of utilizing our bodies as we age can have a profound effect on the development of dry eye. Even a simple loss of eye-hand coordination or a fear of falling may affect personal care. If severe dry eye develops or is already present in an older person, that patient may have lost functional vision and could become further disoriented. As a result of impaired vision, we may not be able to take proper care of ourselves—from performing the most basic everyday activities (dressing ourselves, feeding ourselves) to caring for ourselves medically. If we are unable to see properly, we won't be able to comply with directions from our physician, including reading the contents or directions on a bottle and measuring proper dosage. This scenario may sound extreme, but it happens, and the impact can be dire.

Because dry eye is much more likely to develop as we age, it is imperative that we watch for it in ourselves and in our aging loved ones. If symptoms appear, see a doctor immediately, before the problems intrude seriously on your life or the life of your loved one.

Many diseases and disorders either directly cause dry eye or are closely related to its development. These include Sjögren's syndrome, lupus, rheumatoid arthritis, stroke, diabetes, Graves' and other thyroid-related diseases, and a number of eye disorders. What is interesting about many of these diseases is that they often develop as part of the aging process.

In addition, a number of ailments commonly considered "geriatric diseases," while not technically causes of dry eye, may have a profound impact on the development or treatment of dry eye in an aging or elderly person. Included are Parkinson's disease, osteoarthritis, and various eye disorders including macular degeneration and glaucoma.

### Parkinson's Disease

Common among older people, particularly men, Parkinson's disease is a neurological disorder that results from damage to the part of the brain known as the basal ganglia. The characteristic symptoms include tremors, slow movements, overall stiffness, slurred speech, and a shaky, unbalanced walk. Parkinson's patients often complain of impaired vision and have difficulty reading. The disease may begin as a slight tremor in one hand or arm, but over a period of years affects the entire body. The intellect is usually not altered, but dementia may set in late in the disease.

Although Parkinson's is not a direct cause of dry eye, it may include a dysfunctional autonomic nervous system, which in turn may lead to reduced tear secretion and dry eye. Another symptom is a fixed, unblinking gaze, and the dramatically reduced blink rate may also lead to dry eye. Some tests indicate that patients with Parkinson's disease exhibit reduced androgen levels, which as noted above may also lead to dry eye.

Further, dry eye may be exacerbated by medications taken for Parkinson's disease. Because of difficulty in caring for themselves, these patients have problems coping with other disorders such as anterior blepharitis. When individuals are unable to perform the recommended treatment, relatively benign problems such as blepharitis can quickly evolve into more severe dry eye.

## Arthritis

Dry eye syndrome is closely related to arthritis, especially rheumatoid arthritis, a severe autoimmune disorder that affects the joints and surrounding tissues. When rheumatoid arthritis occurs together with Sjögren's syndrome, as it commonly does, the lacrimal glands are attacked by the immune system and the result is tear-deficient dry eye.

Many patients with dry eye suffer from osteoarthritis (also known as degenerative arthritis), which is the most common type of arthritis that afflicts older people. Osteoarthritis often begins to develop in middle age and can become extremely painful and bothersome as a person ages. Although this form of arthritis is far less serious than rheumatoid arthritis and does not directly cause dry eye, it can affect an older person who already suffers from dry eye. Osteoarthritis affects the joints of the hands and arms, making it very challenging to open bottles and jars, perform eyelid hygiene, or administer eyedrops and other medications to oneself or others. Inserting or removing contact lenses and caring for them properly, and other everyday actions, become problematic and sometimes impossible.

## Other Eye Diseases

Many eye diseases are commonly associated with older patients, especially cataracts, glaucoma, and macular degeneration. Whereas these diseases do not directly cause dry eye syndrome, certain of their aspects may considerably exacerbate existing dry eye.

First, because sight is reduced by any of these disorders, patients tend to stare or gaze intently in an attempt to simply see better. These efforts cause decreased blink rate and exposure, which may lead to dry eye.

Second, these diseases can be incredibly discouraging and depressing. Patients often believe that once they have decreased vision with known moderate glaucoma or macular degeneration, they must accept the irreversibility of this loss of sight. Yet significant dry eye may also be present and affecting the ability to see. Often, attention by both patient and doctor is given to the primary eye disease, while the dry eye may be overlooked and go untreated. If dry eye is also present and is treated, vision may be dramatically improved.

## Geriatric Medications

Most elderly people take medication of some kind. Whether it is for heart disease, depression, Parkinson's, glaucoma, or another disorder, the medication itself may cause or exacerbate dry eye. Here are a few of the common culprits:

- Diuretics (commonly used for heart disease)
- Antihistamines, decongestants (allergies)
- Antipsychotics, antidepressants (depression)
- Antiandrogens (prostate cancer)
- Hormone replacement therapy
- Sleeping pills

It is crucial that you inform your eye doctor of any and all medications you are taking, even over-the-counter medications or herbal remedies. If you have dry eye and require certain medications (as for heart disease or depression), you obviously must continue taking them. Together with your doctor, you need to work therapeutically around the medications to determine that you receive the minimally necessary dosage, but at the same time keep dry eye under control.

Also, be sure you understand how to administer any medi-

BOX 11

**Vision as a Layered Phenomenon**

"Vision as a layered phenomenon" is an expression I have coined to describe the situation when a patient suffers not only from a serious vision-threatening disease such as glaucoma or macular degeneration, but also from an inadequately treated case of dry eye. The fact is that if dry eye is treated with standard treatments, the vision in someone suffering from a more serious vision problem like macular degeneration or glaucoma may be improved (in some cases dramatically). Certainly, the degree of visual loss caused by the dryness may be reversed.

For example, a patient may be suffering from a severe loss of vision due to both macular degeneration and dry eye. If his dry eye problems are reversed, he can go from being unable to see the big E on the eye chart to being able to read a few lines, and from being completely dependent on a spouse or medical helper to being able to dress himself, feed himself, and even prepare meals for himself.

Because the eye is so complex, loss of vision can occur in a number of different ways or layers. If one of the layers can be treated—particularly severe dry eye—vision can be substantially improved.

cation, whether for yourself or for someone in your care. One of my patients suffered from a recurrent corneal infection that we simply could not get under control. We would treat it, then the infection would return. Finally I asked the patient (and his wife) to show me how he put drops in his eyes. It turned out that his wife placed the drops on his forehead, by the nose, then moved his head around so that the drops would roll over his skin into his eyes. In the process, the medication was picking up all the infectious microbes on the surface of his skin and spreading them into his eyes, causing the recurrent infection. Once the couple learned how to properly administer the drops, the infection cleared up quickly and did not recur.

### Administering Eyedrops or Ointments

If you are responsible for the care of an aging relative, it is important that you be vigilant about checking for potential dry eye. Question your relative carefully, if possible, about her vision and potential pain or irritation relating to the eyes. Specifically, look out for classic dry eye signs, including redness around the eye and eyelid, constant watering of the eyes, sensitivity to light, and discharge around the eyes or crustiness on the lids. Because your aging relative or loved one may be incapacitated, even mildly, you may have to administer eyedrops or ointments yourself. It actually is not as difficult as it may appear.

First and foremost, always wash your hands. Ask the patient to lie down or sit with her head tilted back, chin toward the ceiling. With your fingers, draw the lower eyelid down, and ask the patient to look upward. Place a drop or about a half-inch bead of ointment in the sac. Do not touch the cornea or eyelid or lashes with the tube or the dropper tip. Ask the patient to close her eyes, then with a tissue gently remove any excess drops from around the eye. Blot, do not rub. In the case of ointment, if you hold the tube in your hand for a few minutes, your body heat will warm the ointment so it will disperse better over the eye.

Aging and dry eye go together. We may not yet be able to alter the aging process and hormonal changes, but we can anticipate the onset of dry eye. By being proactive, we can reduce its effect on our well-being and thereby age more gracefully.

CHAPTER

# 6

# Allergies, Toxicities, and Other Sensitivities

Myth

*Allergies and dry eye are one and the same.*

Fact

*Allergies and dry eye are very different, but they can overlap and one can cause the other.*

Ocular allergies are commonly encountered by allergists and eye doctors. Statistics vary, but it is fair to say that 50 percent of Americans have some type of allergy, and about 20 percent of Americans (more than 50 million people!) suffer from some sort of allergy that affects the eyes. Since more than 9 million Americans suffer from moderate to severe dry eye (with figures going as high as 20 to 30 million for mild cases), it seems reasonable to surmise that the two often coexist. And, unfortunately, they do. Indeed, some people think ocular allergies and dry eye are the same thing. Many people who suffer from dry eye also develop chronic allergies, while many allergy sufferers, for various reasons, end up with dry eye.

It's important to examine allergies, especially eye-related allergies, because they not only affect your quality of sight, but they can play an enormous role in your quality of life. Allergies can dictate where you live, what you eat, and even how you raise your children (either because they have allergies, or because allergies are frequently hereditary). Obviously, eye allergies can affect your productivity at work, and certainly they can play a part in your choice and enjoyment of leisure activities. Introduce dry eye into the mix, and the situation can quickly become serious.

## THE ALLERGIC REACTION

Generally speaking, an allergy—or an allergic reaction—is a hypersensitivity to a normally harmless substance. The immune system, which includes antibodies, white blood cells, mast cells, and other substances, defends the body against foreign substances called antigens. However, in some people the immune system overresponds to certain antigens (shellfish, peanuts, pollen, grass, cat dander, penicillin) that don't bother other people at all, causing an allergic reaction. In other words, the antigen becomes an allergen, because it incites an allergic reaction.

The immune system, when first exposed to an allergen, has a complicated chemical response. Simply put, it produces a type of antibody called immunoglobulin E (IgE), which binds to certain white blood cells in the blood stream called basophils and to similar cells in the tissues called mast cells. When this now-sensitized person subsequently encounters the allergen, the cells that have IgE on their surface release substances (including histamine) that generate swelling or inflammation in the surrounding tissue. These substances begin a series of reactions that cause ongoing irritation and damage to tissues.

Allergic reactions can be mild to severe. Mild reactions involve watery, itchy eyes; a runny nose; itchy skin; sneezing; hives; and rash. More serious responses include attacks of asthma or an anaphylactic reaction (an extremely severe allergic reaction characterized by a drop in blood pressure and problems with breathing), which can be life threatening.

Because an allergic reaction is triggered by a specific allergen, the allergen needs to be identified in order for the allergy to be reliably alleviated or prevented.

BOX 12

**The Importance of Mast Cells**

Mast cells are central to the ocular allergic process. They are found in connective tissue (for example, the lungs, conjunctiva, nasal, and other mucous membranes) and contain numerous packets of substances (such as histamine) that are released in response to injury or inflammation of bodily tissues. When these substances are released, they are said to degranulate. (For example, simple rubbing of the eye can degranulate mast cells, releasing histamine, which causes the allergic response.) Many medications for allergy or dry eye contain antihistamines to counteract the histamines released from the mast cells. Also, many medications contain mast cell stabilizing agents, which stabilize the mast cells in order to reduce degranulation and histamine release.

## TYPES OF OCULAR ALLERGIES

The term "ocular allergy" refers to a variety of hypersensitivity disorders that affect the eyelid, cornea, and most commonly the conjunctiva. Allergic conjunctivitis breaks down into six groups: seasonal conjunctivitis, perennial conjunctivitis, contact conjunctivitis, giant papillary conjunctivitis (which usually relates to contact lens use); atopic keratoconjunctivitis, and vernal keratoconjunctivitis.

### Seasonal Conjunctivitis

Also known as "hay fever conjunctivitis," because hay fever is a common symptom, seasonal conjunctivitis is the most frequent form of ocular allergy. It involves a response to allergens released in the air at certain times of the year, especially in spring, but also in summer and fall. These include tree pollens (early spring), grasses (usually May through July), weed pollen (August through October), and outdoor molds and decaying leaves. The specific allergens and the timing of their release depend on the geographical area, with warm, dry regions aggravating the problem, since responses tend to start earlier and last longer. Symptoms of seasonal conjunctivitis include itching, tingling, burning, tearing, swollen lids, and sensitivity to light (photophobia), usually in both eyes simultaneously.

### Perennial Conjunctivitis

Whereas seasonal conjunctivitis occurs only at certain times of year, perennial conjunctivitis can be present all year round. In other words, you are supersensitive to certain allergens at any time, not just during a given season. Common perennial allergens include animal danders, dust mites, plant dust, indoor molds, cockroaches (and pesticide sprays!), cotton, and feathers. Symptoms include swollen eyelids, tearing, and redness and itching, also usually in both eyes simultaneously.

### Contact Conjunctivitis

Contact conjunctivitis is a common allergic response to an allergen that has been directly introduced into the eye, like an eyedrop or a cosmetic. The response usually occurs within forty-eight hours of exposure. Itching and tearing of the eye are prevalent, but eczema, swelling, and redness on the eyelid may also be present. Contact conjunctivitis is closely related to contact dermatitis.

### Giant Papillary Conjunctivitis

Giant papillary conjunctivitis (or GPC) is most frequently a disorder of people who wear contact lenses. (It also affects those with ocular prostheses, or those with a history of eye surgery with exposed sutures or other surgical materials.) Symptoms include itching (even after removal of the problematic contact lenses), redness, blurred vision, a foreign body sensation, and excessive mucosal secretions. It also features "giant papillae," which are actually bumps of swollen tissue with a central dilated vessel on the lining of the upper eyelid. In any case, comfortable contact lens wear is just about impossible.

The disorder is usually an allergic-type response to protein deposits on contact lenses, very often soft contact lenses. Sometimes GPC can occur as a reaction to the presence of a lens itself, possibly with an additional toxic or allergic reaction to the lens solutions used for cleaning, disinfecting, or wetting. Regular enzyme treatments for the lenses and proper contact lens cleaning techniques may reduce the chance of GPC. The use of preservative-free solutions can help as well. Once GPC develops, the use of contact lenses usually must be temporarily discontinued until the condition resolves (see also Chapter 7).

## Atopic Keratoconjunctivitis

Atopic keratoconjunctivitis is a chronic, severe, possibly even sight-threatening, condition. Atopic disease is a hereditary disorder, with high levels of IgE antibodies in the blood, marked by the tendency to develop an immediate and strong allergic reaction to substances such as pollen, certain foods, and animal dander. It can manifest as hay fever, asthma, eczema, or similar allergic conditions.

The disorder usually begins in middle age (30–50) and generally affects men. It occurs with atopic dermatitis, and together they inflame the eyelids, conjunctiva, and cornea. This is a perennial allergy that affects both eyes simultaneously. Symptoms may include tearing, burning, and itching of the eyes, together with thick, abundant secretions. With advanced atopic keratoconjunctivitis, scarring of the cornea and blindness may occur.

### Vernal Keratoconjunctivitis

This rare disorder may also affect the cornea with scarring and ingrown blood vessels and is most often seen in dry, hot climates or areas with high incidence of air pollution. It usually appears in boys under the age of 10 with a genetic history of allergy, although it often stabilizes in adulthood or progresses to atopic keratoconjunctivitis. Symptoms include severe itching, a foreign body sensation, tearing, and photophobia.

### Related Allergies

A number of common allergies—particularly rhinitis (nasal allergy), dermatitis (skin allergies), and asthma (allergy of the breathing airways)—are closely related to ocular allergies, and by association to dry eye. Frequently, my dry eye patients suffer from one or more of these allergies.

Allergic rhinitis is inflammation and swelling of the mucous membrane of the nose, characterized by a runny nose and stuffiness. Many—if not most—people with allergic rhinitis have ocular allergy as well, typically seasonal and perennial conjunctivitis. The condition is caused by reaction of the body's immune system to environmental triggers: dust, molds, pollens, grasses, trees, or animals. Symptoms include sneezing, runny nose, stuffiness, and itchy, watery eyes. Often the patient has a family history of allergies. Avoiding the substance that triggers the allergy prevents symptoms, but often avoidance isn't possible.

Prescription nasal steroids and antihistamine sprays can be used to treat allergic rhinitis. Oral antihistamines (like Benadryl) will dry out the mucous membrane of the nose, but also cause sleepiness and dry eye. It is important to note that you may control a nasal allergy with eyedrops, but you can't control an eye allergy with a nasal spray. In other words, eye treatments can drip into the nose, but nose treatments do not work their way up to the eye. Therefore, although allergic rhinitis and allergic conjunctivitis often appear together, they may need to be treated separately.

Dermatitis (or eczema) refers to an inflammation of the upper layers of the skin, causing itching, blisters, redness, swelling and often oozing, scabbing, and scaling. Some types of dermatitis affect only specific parts of the body, whereas others can occur anywhere; some types have a known cause, others do not. Dermatitis is always the skin's way of reacting to a substance that is causing irritation or an allergy. Although sometimes the allergen is swallowed, usually it comes in direct contact with the skin. This is called allergic contact dermatitis. It often appears as a rash and is caused by the skin's direct contact with a particular substance, such as poison ivy, a metal, or a cosmetic. The rash is very itchy, is confined to a specific area, and frequently has clearly defined boundaries. Dermatitis may be a brief reaction to a particular substance, or it may be chronic and persist over time.

Asthma is a condition in which the airways (including the mouth, throat, windpipe, and lungs) are swollen and narrowed because of hypersensitivity to certain stimuli, including pollen, dust mites, animal dander, smoke, and even cold air and exercise. In an asthma attack, the smooth muscles of the bronchi go into spasm, and the tissues lining the airways swell and secrete mucus into the airways. These actions narrow the diameter of the airways (a condition called bronchoconstriction), and the sufferer has trouble breathing. Asthma attacks vary in frequency and severity. Some people with asthma are symptom free most of the time, with an occasional brief episode of shortness of breath. Others cough or wheeze most of the time and have severe attacks after colds, exercise, or exposure to allergies. Even crying or laughing may bring on symptoms.

Asthma is a serious disease and can be fatal. Closely associated with atopic disease, it is often evident in patients with atopic keratoconjunctivitis. Treatment includes oral antihistamines, which with chronic use can lead to dry eye, or if dry eye is already present, can exacerbate the problem.

BOX 13

**Contact Dermatitis and Your Eyes**

Contact dermatitis, or skin allergies, can be caused by any number of things. It is important to be aware of them, because it is easy to transport an allergen from the skin to the eyelid and even to the surface of the eye, just by everyday rubbing of the eyes. Here are a few examples of common skin allergens. If you are susceptible to contact dermatitis, the best treatment is simply to avoid the allergen. To protect your eyes, keep your fingers away from your eyes and face!

*Plants:* poison ivy, poison oak, poison sumac, ragweed, dried leaves, houseplants

*Metals* (in jewelry, on handles of tools, etc.): nickel, chromium, cobalt

*Cosmetics:* nail polish; nail polish remover; deodorants; moisturizers; aftershave; perfumes, colognes, and other fragrances; sunscreens; eye makeup (mascara, liner, eye shadow); face powder, hair sprays and dyes

*Chemicals used in clothing:* rubber, especially latex (used by doctors and dentists) in gloves, shoes, undergarments, other apparel; dry cleaning chemicals; laundry detergent

*Cleaning products:* ammonia, bleach, strong soaps and detergents, drain cleaners, cleaning sprays, oven cleaner

*Drugs:* antibiotics; prescription ointments, creams, and lotions (even some used to treat dermatitis); novocaine

BOX 14

**Looks Can Be Deceiving**

Sometimes eyelids can become irritated with eczema and end up creating a situation—itching, redness, a foreign body sensation—that looks very much like dry eye. Recently, a 50-year-old glaucoma specialist complained to me of a burning and foreign body sensation in his right eye. He had tried to treat the problem using over-the-counter artificial tears for dry eye, but with no effect. I took a look and realized that he had a subtle case of eczema on his eyelid. I prescribed a mild steroid ophthalmic ointment that he applied directly to the lid, and the problem cleared up overnight.

## CHRONIC ALLERGIES

If you or someone in your home suffers from chronic allergies (especially asthma), here are a few precautions you can take to keep common household allergens (including dust mites, molds, feathers, cockroaches, animal dander) to a minimum. These precautions are also applicable to dry eye sufferers:

Invest in an air purifier or HEPA (High Efficiency Particulate Arrestance) air cleaner to keep the household air free of dander, pollen, pollutants, and other allergens.

Change air-conditioning vent filters frequently, and make sure heating equipment is vented properly. Keep windows closed as much as possible. Use outdoor venting fans in the kitchen, bath, and laundry areas (to pull air out of the house), but avoid window or attic fans (which may pull allergen-laden air into the house).

Remove all wall-to-wall carpets; instead use hardwood, vinyl, linoleum tile, or slate flooring. If you must have carpets or rugs, choose low pile.

If you keep any carpets or rugs, steam clean or wash in hot water frequently. Vacuum with a low-emission vacuum cleaner with a HEPA filter.

Remove shoes when you enter the house to avoid tracking in outdoor allergens.

Avoid having pets, especially cats and dogs. If you already have pets, keep them out of the house, or at a minimum bar them from the bedrooms.

Keep the relative humidity in the house low (below 50 percent, unless dry eye is a problem, in which case keep it at 50 percent). Avoid damp rooms like cellars and basements. Use a dehumidifier, if necessary.

Prohibit cigarette, cigar, or pipe smoking in the house.

Avoid burning a fire in your fireplace, and avoid burning candles and incense.

Avoid scented products including candles, incense, air fresheners, and scented cleaners.

Remove all houseplants.

Use special antiallergic (mite proof) pillow cases and mattress covers.

Keep your home cockroach free.

Wash all laundry in hottest water possible. Dry clothes in a dryer; don't hang them outdoors where pollen and other allergens can collect on them.

Fix leaks that allow mold to grow.

Clean moldy surfaces in showers or under sinks.

Reduce dust by eliminating clutter.

## OCULAR ALLERGIES AND DRY EYE

Because allergic conjunctivitis and dry eye are both common conditions with similar symptoms, they may cause confusion and misdiagnosis. In fact, dry eye is frequently mistaken for

BOX 15

**Pet Allergies—But No Pet?**

A recent study found that nearly every home in the sample tested positive for pet allergies, although less than half of the homes actually had a pet. It turned out that cat and dog dander was brought into the home on the clothing and shoes of family members. A child might have played with a friend's cat, or an adult might have casually petted a neighbor's dog passing on the street. What was even more surprising was that the dander made its way into the house in sufficient quantities to cause an allergic response.

allergic conjunctivitis, and often patients suffer from both problems at the same time without knowing it.

To diagnose whether you have allergy or dry eye, you can perform a couple of simple tests. The rule of thumb is, "If it itches, it's an allergy; if it scratches, it's dry eye." In other words, if allergens are on the eye, the eye will itch—rather like a mosquito bite itches. If the tear glands are not operating properly and the eye is dry, the eye will feel scratchy, as though a foreign body is present.

Another helpful test is the maximum blink-interval test. Look straight ahead, keeping your eyes open, and count the seconds until you feel a burning sensation in your eyes. If more than seven seconds elapse before you need to blink, you're fine; if less than seven seconds pass, you may well have dry eye. (If less than five seconds pass, you almost certainly have dry eye!)

## How One Leads to the Other

Not only are ocular allergies and dry eye different, one can cause the other—or at least make the other worse.

If you suffer from an allergy that affects your eyes (hay fever or other seasonal allergy, an allergy to pet dander, a contact allergy to eye makeup), it can turn into dry eye. Here's how: The allergic reaction releases histamine and other inflammatory mediators from the mast cells onto the eyes, which disrupts both the mucin and the lipid phases, and directly alters tear film quality, shortening the tear breakup time. The result is dry eye symptoms that may persist for weeks after the allergic episode. If the inflammation becomes chronic, changes may occur, including lid swelling and obstructive meibomian gland dysfunction as well as goblet cell loss with mucin deficiency—in other words, evaporative dry eye. Chronic inflammation numbs the ocular surface, thereby affecting the lacrimal functional unit, which can result in aqueous tear deficient dry eye as well.

To compound the problem, allergies are often treated with pills that contain antihistamines. The antihistamines relieve the allergic symptoms but dry out the mucous membrane and cause or exacerbate dry eye.

On the other hand, dry eye can exacerbate, and even create, allergies. If you have dry eye, tears are not washing allergens out of the eye. And the allergens are of higher concentration because they are not being adequately diluted with tears. As a result, if you have dry eye and also suffer from allergies, both your dry eye and your allergies can become worse!

Finally, you can have ocular allergy (or allergies) and dry eye at the same time. Both are chronic conditions, with symptoms that may be intermittent yet overlap.

## When the Cure Is the Culprit

Treatment for dry eye accompanied by allergies can be a real problem. As we've discussed, common seasonal or perennial allergies frequently are treated with pills (including over-the-counter allergy pills like Benadryl or Tylenol PM, or prescription medications like Zyrtec or Claritin) as well as eyedrops and nasal sprays that contain antihistamines that dry out the ocular surface. In other words, dry eye can be aggravated or caused by use of these common over-the-counter allergy medications.

Artificial tears and other therapeutic eyedrops pose additional problems for people with both ocular allergies and dry eye. A number of over-the-counter eyedrops and liquid tears contain preservatives, and many people are allergic or sensitive to those preservatives or develop allergies over time. (Specifically, the preservatives can be toxic to the epithelial cells on the conjunctiva and cornea, and some can dissolve the lipid tear layer through a detergent effect. Preservatives in artificial tears or eyedrops can also build up on contact lenses, resulting in an allergic or toxic effect.)

Another problematic element in many eyedrops is the presence of vasoconstrictors, chemicals used to constrict blood vessels in order to remove redness from inflamed eyes. Common over-the-counter products such as Visine ("get the red out") or Naphcon-A contain these chemicals. They are problematic because they may mask other symptoms, as well as possibly decrease tear production because of reduced blood flow to the tear glands.

The bottom line is that medications designed to treat ocular allergies may exacerbate dry eye. What's more, products created to alleviate dry eye pain may have the opposite effect, because the preservatives and vasoconstrictors in the medications may be toxic and sting the eyes. In some cases, the cure is worse than the problem.

## Treating Ocular Allergies and Dry Eye

If you are suffering from either ocular allergies and/or dry eye (see Box 16), you can adopt a few simple remedies to ease your eye pain. All the medications suggested here are available over the counter. (For more information about treatment, see Chapter 10.)

BOX 16

**Do You Have Dry Eye or an Ocular Allergy?**

**A Self-Test**

**1** *Do your eyes itch? Or do your eyes feel scratchy, gritty, or sandy?*
If they itch, it's an allergy; if they feel scratchy or gritty, it's dry eye.

**2** *Do you pass the maximum blink-interval test? Can you keep your eyes open for at least seven seconds before feeling a burning sensation?*
If you can keep your eyes open without blinking for at least seven seconds, you can be fairly certain that you don't have dry eye. If you experienced eye pain in less than seven seconds, you may have dry eye.

**3** *Do other members of your family have symptoms similar to yours, or suffer from hay fever, asthma, eczema, or motion sickness?*
If other members of your family have a similar problem, it is probably an allergy. Allergies are often hereditary.

**4** *Do your symptoms show up at specific times of year, particularly in the spring or fall?*
If the symptoms show up at a particular time of year, especially in the spring or summer or fall, you are likely to have a seasonal allergy. You are probably sensitive to various pollens, grasses, leaves, or trees.

**5** *Do you have symptoms when you enter a house having a cat or dog?*
If you experience itchy eyes when you are around house pets, you probably have an allergy to pet dander.

**6** *Do your symptoms get progressively worse as the day wears on?*
If your eyes get scratchier or burn more later in the day, you may well have dry eye. Eyes tend to get more dry and irritated the longer you use them without rest.

**7** *Are your eyelids swollen and red?*
If so, you probably have an allergy. Swollen, red eyelids are typically related to allergic dermatitis and are not normally a symptom of dry eye.

**8** *Does irrigation of your eye with eye rinse reduce symptoms?*
If your eyes are dramatically, if only temporarily, soothed after using an eye rinse, you probably have an allergy. Eye rinses, which wash away allergens, are saline solutions, not lubricants, and typically will not significantly improve dry eye.

**9** *Does a blink improve your vision momentarily?*
If the answer is yes, you probably have dry eye. A blink spreads tears over the ocular surface, and if your eyes are dry, your vision will improve. If you have an allergy without dry eye, a blink will not enhance your vision because you already have adequate tears. Vision improves only momentarily, because the eye becomes dry again.

**10** *Does an artificial tear improve your vision momentarily?*
Once more, if the answer is yes, you probably have dry eye. The artificial tear enhances vision if the eye is dry, but the effect will last only until the eye is dry again.

Identify and, if possible, remove allergens from your home: plants, pets, household chemicals, and the like. If you have seasonal allergies, prepare for them.

Keep your hands away from your eyes, and wash them frequently. If you rub your eyes, you may be transporting allergens to your eyes, squeezing mast cells, and thus releasing more histamines. No more rubbing!

Lubricate your eyes frequently with artificial tears. Refrigerating them beforehand will increase your relief. However, make sure you select tears that do not contain preservatives. Also, avoid drops that promise to remove redness.

Irrigate your eyes with over-the-counter sterile ophthalmic saline, which may help wash out unwanted allergens.

Try cold compresses for relief.

Remember that if you have serious dry eye syndrome as well as chronic allergies, you need to work closely with your eye doctor to be sure you get optimal relief.

CHAPTER

# 7

# Contact Lenses

Myth

*Long-term contact lens wear can improve your vision.*

Fact

*Long-term contact lens wear can inhibit the sensation on your cornea, leading to various vision problems, including dry eye.*

Problems with contact lens wear are a hallmark of dry eye syndrome and, not surprisingly, dry eye is one of the most common complaints of contact lens wearers. It would be safe to say that the majority of patients who come into my office wearing contact lenses and experiencing chronic pain and irritation are likely to be diagnosed with dry eye syndrome.

Contact lens wear and dry eyes create an interesting relationship in that the wearing of the contact lens—a foreign body—requires a greater volume of tears for the lenses to work properly. Ironically, however, the long-term presence of contact lenses can lead to decreased tear volume and dry eye.

## ABOUT CONTACT LENSES

Contact lenses are one of the most common ways to correct simple refractive vision problems, and because of advances in technology, contact lens use has increased exponentially over the past twenty years or so. Unfortunately, so has dry eye syndrome, and it would appear that the two phenomena are related.

A contact lens is a specially shaped plastic disk that sits on the cornea of your eye—in more or less direct contact with the eye. Actually, a contact lens floats on the eye's natural tears. The outer and inner surfaces of each lens are ground to fit the curvature of the eye and correct a particular refraction problem, including nearsightedness, farsightedness, and, with newer types of lenses, astigmatism and presbyopia. People choose contact lenses to improve the quality of vision, to derive greater comfort, and because they believe lenses will make them more attractive than spectacles. Besides, some patients have occupational needs that are incompatible with glasses. However, contact lenses (especially soft lenses) require greater attention to hygiene and care than regular glasses, and occasionally contact lenses can damage the eye. Allergies, infection, and dry eye syndrome can result.

Contact lenses are most suitable for people with ordinary refractive problems: nearsightedness, farsightedness, astigmatism, and in some special circumstances, after cornea transplants. Because insertion and care of contact lenses require a degree of manual dexterity, they are probably not advisable for young children or elderly people, especially those suffering with dexterity problems from arthritis or Parkinson's disease. Also, contact lenses may not be appropriate for those who suffer from frequent and chronic allergies or from severe dry eye. An exception may be a relatively new prosthetic device called the Boston scleral lens, which has been developed for people with severe ocular surface diseases, including dry eye, who do not respond to other treatments. This lens is a fluid-ventilated gas-permeable contact lens that rests entirely on the sclera (the white of the eye), creating a fluid-filled space over the diseased cornea.

## TYPES OF LENSES

Two types of contact lenses are readily available today: rigid gas-permeable (RGP) lenses (small, firm plastic disks that fit over part of the cornea) and soft lenses (thin, flexible polymer disks that generally sit over a larger portion of the eye and cover the entire cornea.) The old-fashioned, so-called hard lenses, also known as PMMA lenses, are rarely prescribed these days.

### Rigid Gas-Permeable Lenses

Rigid gas-permeable lenses have pores in the plastic that allow oxygen to reach the cornea, increasing the comfort of lens wear. RGP lenses are easier to care for than soft lenses in that they don't tear, although they may occasionally crack. Rigid lenses have long been prescribed to people with astigmatism, because the lens creates a smooth optical surface and makes vision clearer. (However, the newer toric lenses are allowing people with astigmatism to wear soft lenses.)

Initially, rigid lenses are less comfortable to wear than soft lenses, and it may take several days of measured wear to get used to them. They also tend to slide around on the eye more readily than soft lenses. However, many people believe that their vision is sharper with rigid lenses and for that reason prefer them. Rigid lenses can last for several years, thus are more economical over the long term.

### Soft Lenses

Soft lenses are generally the lenses-of-choice over rigid lenses. Because the polymer plastic from which they are made is thinner, more flexible, and causes less friction on the eye, soft lenses are far more comfortable to wear. While adjusting to rigid lenses takes several days, soft lenses can be worn virtually immediately and tend to float (stay) on the eye better.

Soft lenses come in a number of "formats," including conventional daily reusable soft lenses, disposable soft lenses, extended-wear reusable lenses, and toric lenses for astigmatism.

Conventional daily reusable soft lenses are the most common type of soft lens, and should last, with proper care, for about a year.

Disposable lenses are soft lenses that are designed to be discarded daily or on a two-week basis, depending on the type. They are an appropriate choice for people who suffer from allergies, in that the problem of allergen and other deposit buildup on the lenses is vastly reduced. On the other hand, disposable lenses are more expensive, by the mere fact that they are regularly thrown away. Users sometimes wear the lenses longer than the recommended one day (or two weeks), increasing the risk of allergic reaction.

For former contact lens wearers who are being treated for allergies with or without dry eye, I recommend that they resume contact lens wear by using daily disposable contact lenses.

Extended-wear reusable lenses are designed to be worn for longer lengths of time (seven to thirty days, depending on the type, including during sleep). They are thinner than conventional soft lenses, making them more comfortable but also more fragile.

Recently, thirty-day wear contacts made a comeback. Extended-wear lenses originally came on the market in the early 1980s, but many professionals decided that overnight use was too risky, leading to conjunctivitis, infectious cornea ulcers, and more serious problems. However, in 2001 the Food and Drug Administration approved a new type of extended-wear lens made of superpermeable silicone hydrogel. This lens is superior to the older type of extended-wear lens because it is able to provide more oxygen to the cornea. Examples include "Focus Night & Day" by CIBA Vision and "Pure Vision" by Bausch and Lomb.

With these new lenses, many people are able to use extended-wear lenses continuously for days (or weeks) with greater comfort and safety. But sleeping in contact lenses still increases the risk for various problems including conjunctivitis, corneal infection with ulceration and possible blindness.

Therefore, if you use extended-wear lenses, exercise extreme caution. Because the new silicone hydrogel lenses allow better oxygen transmission to the cornea, I do endorse them. However, I recommend that all soft lenses be worn *only* on a daily-wear basis. Remove the lenses immediately and see your eye doctor if you experience any sign of persistent eye redness, pain, blurred vision, or sensitivity to light.

### Toric Lenses

Toric lenses are specially designed for people who suffer from astigmatism. To correct astigmatism effectively, the lens must rest on the eye securely in a precise orientation. Often with astigmatism, when you blink, the lens rotates slightly, causing blurred or fluctuating vision. Toric lenses are designed to ensure minimal movement and return to the correct orientation, assuring continuous stability of vision.

### Other Types

These days, manufacturers of contact lenses are coming up with a wide range of lenses to cover a variety of vision problems. In addition to the toric lenses for those with astigmatism, bifocals or monovision lenses are available for people with presbyopia; special tinted lenses are on the market for cosmetic purposes; and ultraviolet-blocking contacts are useful for people who work or play outdoors in harsh sunlight.

As mentioned earlier, the Boston scleral lens is now used for those with cornea diseases, including severe dry eye, who are not responding to conventional therapies. In addition, contacts are being developed for people who live or work in dry environments, travel frequently in airplanes or automobiles, sit in front of computers for long periods, or are frequently exposed to dry heat or air conditioning. Time will tell if these innovations will help reduce the incidence or impact of dry eye.

## CARING FOR YOUR LENSES

An overwhelming array of products is available in most drugstores or supermarkets for the care of contact lenses. Despite the number of products, contact lens care these days is easier than ever.

## Caring for Rigid Lenses

Rigid lenses require special care, and solutions designed especially for the care of RGPs should be used. The lenses should be cleaned and rinsed daily to remove oils, cosmetics, and other debris, then stored overnight in a disinfecting-conditioning solution to kill microorganisms and keep the lens flexible. They may require periodic enzymatic cleaning. If you have sensitive eyes, you should look for preservative-free solutions.

Here's how rigid lenses should be cleaned:

1. Place the lenses one at a time in the palm of your hand, and put a few drops of detergent-based lens cleaner on them. Rub in a circular motion with your index finger for twenty to thirty seconds.
2. Rinse with a commercial contact lens saline solution.
3. Place in a rigid contact lens storage-disinfection solution for at least four hours (or as recommended by the manufacturer).
4. Rinse with a sterile solution and/or add a wetting solution, as desired.
5. Insert the contacts into your eye.

For enzyme cleaning, clean your lenses first with the daily cleaner, then allow the lenses to soak in the enzyme solution for at least two hours. Clean and disinfect the lenses before returning them to your eyes.

Because rigid lenses last longer than soft lenses (often for several years) it is crucial to have your lenses checked on your eyes by your eye care practitioner once a year and have them polished as needed to remove scratches.

## Caring for Soft Lenses

With soft lenses, a lens solution should be used every day to remove film and deposits from the lens surface, to disinfect the lenses, and to provide appropriate storage. Excellent multipur-

BOX 17

**General Guidelines for Contact Lens Use**

Here are a few guidelines for users of all types of lenses to ensure safety and health:

Always wash your hands before handling your contacts.
Bear in mind that different solutions are used for soft lenses and for rigid lenses. Be sure you select the correct ones when you are purchasing them, or check with your eye doctor.
Use only sterile, commercially prepared contact lens solutions unless otherwise directed by your eye doctor.
Keep your lens case as clean as your lenses; clean it thoroughly once a week and replace it every month, perhaps when you buy new solutions.
Avoid using solutions after their expiration dates.
Never reuse cleaning or disinfecting solutions.
Never use tap water or saliva to clean lenses.
Never store contacts in nonsterile liquids such as tap water, bottled water, or homemade saline solutions.

pose solutions that can be used to clean, rinse, disinfect, and store lenses are readily available in any drugstore. Together with a periodic enzymatic cleaning, these solutions work very well. (Check the label, however, and make sure that the solution does not contain the preservative thimerosal, which can irritate sensitive eyes.)

If you have very sensitive eyes, I suggest that you use a completely preservative-free system to care for your soft lenses. Such systems normally include the following steps:

1. Clean each lens, one at a time, with a preservative-free cleaner; rinse with preservative-free saline solution.
2. Store the lenses in their storage cup in a preservative-free disinfecting solution (for example, 3 percent hydrogen peroxide), to which a neutralizing tablet has been added four to six hours or overnight.
3. Rinse with a preservative-free saline solution.
4. Add a preservative-free wetting solution, if desired.
5. Insert the contacts into your eyes.

Like rigid lenses, soft lenses should be treated weekly with an enzyme solution to clean off protein. An enzyme tablet can be inserted in the storage cup with the neutralizing tablet. (At the time this book went to press, the safety of multipurpose solutions was being questioned. Ask your eye doctor which are the best lens-care solutions.)

### Caring for the Lens Case

When not in use, your lens case should be rinsed with hot, soapy tap water and dried carefully. Replace your case every month (or whenever you buy new lens solution) to reduce the risk of infection.

## DRY EYE AND CONTACT-LENS ISSUES

Contact lens wear can lead to dry eye for several reasons: problems with the long-term wear, problems relating to the lenses themselves, allergies, and inadequate hygiene.

### Long-Term Wear

Long-term contact lens wear (and many individuals have worn contacts for decades) can result in decreased sensation on the cornea, and, as we know, decreased corneal sensation leads to decreased tear production, decreased blinking, and ultimately full-blown dry eye syndrome.

A contact lens works properly only if it floats easily on an adequate layer of tear film. If the tear film is not wet enough (that is, if the lacrimal glands are not producing sufficient watery tears) or evaporates too quickly, the contact lens will not only fail to correct your vision properly, it will feel incredibly painful on your eye—almost like a salty potato chip.

### The Lenses Themselves

The makeup of the contact lenses themselves can sometimes be responsible for dry eye. Soft contact lenses are made from plastics that contain a substantial amount of water, anywhere from about 25 to 60 percent. The more water a soft contact lens contains, the more prone it is to dehydration, or losing its water. As the water evaporates from the surface of the lens while on the eye, it can cause dehydration on the surface of the eye, ultimately resulting in dry eye. Other indoor or outdoor environmental conditions (heat, wind, smoke) may exacerbate this condition.

Rigid gas-permeable lenses are made of materials that do not contain water. Although at first glance that may appear to be a solution for the dehydration problem, the opposite is true. The polymer that makes up RGP lenses is hydrophobic and tends to repel water, making the surface of the eye more prone to drying.

Both rigid and soft lenses may rub or chafe the surface of the eye, upsetting the tear film stability. Sometimes rigid lenses can nick the cornea, causing pain; or dust, dirt, or other microbes can be caught under the lens, resulting in inflammation and possibly infection.

### Allergies and Inadequate Hygiene

Allergies to contact lenses are usually a response to protein buildup on the lenses due to inadequate hygiene. I say "inadequate hygiene" as opposed to "poor hygiene," because a person may responsibly clean his lenses each day and use enzymes appropriately, but because of personal genetics still accumulate deposits and develop allergies. Also, as with dry eye solutions, some people are allergic to the lens care solution itself.

Giant papillary conjunctivitis is one of the most frequent disorders affecting people who wear contact lenses, and is a type of allergic reaction to protein and lipid deposits on the lenses. It can also be caused by the presence in the eyes of the lenses themselves, or possibly even by the solutions used for lens care. (For a more extended discussion of GPC, see Chapter 6.)

GPC symptoms include itching, redness, blurred vision, a foreign body sensation, and excessive mucosal secretions. The disorder also features "giant papillae," which are actually bumps of swollen tissue with a central dilated vessel on the lining of the upper eyelid. In any case, comfortable contact lens wear is impossible.

To remedy the situation or to help prevent GPC, performing regular (usually at least weekly) enzyme treatments for the lenses, using proper contact lens care techniques, and choosing preservative-free solutions may help. If you have been wearing soft lenses, switching to rigid gas-permeable lenses may prevent GPC, since research has shown that people who wear gas-permeable lenses develop the disorder less frequently. Once GPC develops, the use of contact lenses usually must be temporarily discontinued until the condition is resolved.

## IF YOU SUSPECT YOU HAVE DRY EYE

If you suspect you have dry eye, stop wearing your contact lenses immediately and have your eyes examined by your eye doctor as soon as possible. Otherwise, without even being aware of it, you may end up scarring your cornea; sensation on the corneal surface will have decreased as a result of both the contact lens wear and the chronic dry eye.

If you are suffering from aqueous tear deficient dry eye, you may be treated with artificial tears, a mild topical steroid called Lotemax, or a relatively new eyedrop called Restasis. If you are still not producing enough tears, your eye doctor may suggest a

BOX 18

**Case Study: Erin**

Erin, a 30-year-old woman, came to me with severely inflamed eyes. She had used contact lenses for almost twenty years, since her early teens, wearing soft daily-wear reusable lenses for the past several years. For most of that time she had had no problem, but suddenly she had been experiencing intense pain in her eyes, together with extreme irritation and blurry vision. Her eyes were bright red.

Upon examination, I saw that she had serious corneal problems. Her eyes were inflamed from meibomian gland dysfunction, and blood vessels were growing into her cornea because of the inflammation and dry eye. Given the extent of her difficulties, I could see that the situation had persisted for a long time. Because Erin had worn contacts for so many years, the sensation in her cornea was drastically reduced. As a result, she simply hadn't felt any pain until the problem was acute.

To treat her problems, I discontinued her use of contact lenses. I prescribed a regimen of eyelid hygiene consisting of warm compresses to the eyes and careful cleansing of the lid margins once a day with baby shampoo diluted with tap water. I prescribed tear supplements, mild steroid drops, and oral tetracycline to help decrease the inflammation.

After two months, she was able to resume wearing contacts (silicone hydrogel lenses on a daily-wear basis). Much stricter now in her lid hygiene, she is doing very well.

punctal occlusion, which is a simple closing of the tear duct so that sufficient tears remain on the surface of the eye. If you have evaporative dry eye from meibomian gland dysfunction, your doctor may suggest special therapies including eyedrops, eyelid hygiene, topical and oral anti-inflammatory medication, or nutritional supplements.

The fact that you have dry eye syndrome doesn't mean you can never wear contact lenses again. However, your eye problems should be brought under control before you resume. For people with allergies, consider using daily disposable soft lenses, since contact lenses tend to absorb harmful deposits that cause ocular allergies. Both allergy sufferers and dry eye patients should be scrupulous about contact lens care and usage, and consider using preservative-free lens solutions whenever possible. Meticulous care of your contact lenses and adequate treatment of your dry eye will usually enable you to wear your contacts again.

## MYTH AND REALITY

Many people believe that wearing contact lenses for years will actually improve their vision. This is not true! Part of the reason why the myth is so believable is that when many people remove their contacts, their corneas have warped, retaining the shape of the contact for several hours or longer. Thus they may see well enough to forgo wearing glasses for a brief period. But eventually the corneas will resume their normal shape, whether that means a return to nearsightedness, farsightedness, astigmatism, or a combination of vision problems.

Wearing contacts for several hours each day and especially overnight is actually detrimental to many people, even those using extended-wear lenses, because the eye needs rest and relaxation from the foreign body each and every day. In addition, as we've seen, after contacts have been worn for years, the cornea may become desensitized, which in turn may lead to dry eye syndrome.

CHAPTER

# 8

# LASIK and Other Refractive Surgeries

Myth

*LASIK surgery is a quick and simple procedure to correct refractive vision problems and has nothing to do with dry eye syndrome.*

Fact

*LASIK is a complex operation and problems, especially dry eye, may develop or worsen after the procedure.*

Refractive surgery is used to correct refractive eye problems: nearsightedness, farsightedness, and astigmatism. Many types of refractive surgery have been developed over the past twenty or thirty years, but today the procedures most frequently performed are LASIK (laser in situ keratomileusis), PRK (photorefractive keratectomy), LASEK (laser subepithelial keratomileusis), and epi-LASIK (epithelial laser in situ keratomileusis).

All of these procedures use laser surgery to reshape the cornea, the goal being to focus light directly onto the retina. Ideally, vision is thereby improved to the point where spectacles or contact lenses are no longer needed. In theory, refractive surgery corrects vision to the extent that glasses or contact lenses correct vision, although occasionally it doesn't quite work out that way.

## WHO HAS REFRACTIVE SURGERY AND WHY

According to figures compiled by Jobson Publishing LLC, a firm that specializes in optical industry statistics, about 1.8 million vision-correction (refractive) procedures were performed in 2001. Since most people have refractive surgery in both eyes, this means that about 900,000 people elected to have refractive surgery in 2001. The number was up from about 750,000 in 2000, and from a total of 1.2 million over the preceding three years, or an average of about 400,000 people per year. (The American Academy of Ophthalmology reports similar figures.) The bottom line is that more and more people are electing to have refractive surgery. At the same time, a Gallup poll taken in 2003 revealed that many people still knew little about refractive surgery (particularly LASIK) and were completely unaware of advances in the field.

Most people who elect to have LASIK surgery want to alleviate their dependency on conventional eyeglasses, and especially on contact lenses. Many are tired of the inconvenience of wearing—and taking proper care of—contact lenses, and some resent the dollars spent over the years for replacement lenses and lens care solutions. Some persons, especially those who suffer from dry eye, simply can no longer tolerate wearing their contact lenses. Most are adults in the prime of life (usually between ages 21 and 49), and many are active in sports such as swimming, biking, or skiing—activities that make wearing glasses or contact lenses annoying, if not downright troublesome. A significant number are also interested in the cosmetic advantages of refractive surgery.

In general, LASIK and other refractive surgeries are not recommended for individuals under the age of 18, or for people whose eyeglass prescription has recently changed (especially middle-aged people who are beginning to experience presbyopia). Medically, LASIK is not recommended for people with thin, swollen, flat, or warped corneas; a history of corneal epithelium erosion; dystrophy; or other cornea problems. You should ask your doctor if these issues are a problem for you. Nor is LASIK advisable for people with large pupils, cataracts, glaucoma, chronic allergies, chronic blepharitis, or uncontrolled dry eye. Finally, refractive surgery is generally not suitable for those who suffer from a serious autoimmune disease such as rheumatoid arthritis, lupus, Sjögren's syndrome, or for patients with diabetes.

## THE REFRACTIVE SURGERIES

Many refractive surgeries are available today, but the four most frequently used are LASIK, PRK, LASEK, and epi-LASIK. These are all photoablation laser procedures, which means that a laser is used to permanently reshape the cornea surface. Three of these surgeries involve a flap, or a piece of epithelium (plus, with LASIK, a thin layer of stroma) that is folded back and then replaced after the cornea has been lasered. (PRK does not involve the creation of a flap.)

### LASIK (laser in situ keratomileusis)

LASIK is by far the most popular and the most commonly performed of the various refractive surgeries. Compared to the other types, the postoperative period is less painful, and vision is improved almost immediately. (With PRK, for example, the procedure itself is more painful and the surface of the cornea must heal before vision is restored or improves, a process that may take anywhere from three to seven days for functional vision, and six weeks to six months for complete visual stability.)

Performed on an outpatient basis, the LASIK procedure is completed in about twenty minutes. (The actual surgery usually takes less than one minute.) The patient is awake the entire time, although the doctor may provide a mild oral sedative.

Here's how it is done:

As a patient, you lie down on a cot next to a special instrument called an excimer laser. Your eye is numbed with eyedrops, then is positioned directly under the laser. (One eye is operated on at a time.) An instrument called a speculum is used to keep the eye open, and a suction ring placed over the eye pressurizes it to aid the surgeon.

With a special instrument called a microkeratome, the surgeon cuts a very thin flap in the central part of the cornea, slicing through the epithelium to the corneal stroma. Or the flap can be created with an Intralase laser; in this process, low-level suction is used to hold the eye still while the laser makes the flap. In either case, the flap is then folded back to reveal the deeper corneal tissues. As the patient focuses on a target light, a laser is used to vaporize or ablate a tiny amount of corneal tissue under the flap in order to reshape the cornea. The lasering is experienced as a mild pulsing sensation and is not painful. The stronger your prescription, the more time the surgery will take, but in any case it is only a few minutes. The flap is laid back in place and in some cases a bandage contact lens is applied. You will then rest with your eyes closed for a few minutes before the surgeon operates on the other eye. Many people have both eyes done on the same day, while others allow a week or so to pass between procedures.

Most people experience little pain or discomfort after LASIK surgery, although eyes may be irritated, watery, or light sensitive for a few days afterward. Your vision should improve rapidly, usually in less than twenty-four hours. It should continue to improve and be normally stabilized within six weeks. Although you must have someone to take you home immediately after the surgery, generally you can return to work—and other everyday activities—within one to three days.

### PRK (photorefractive keratectomy)

Generally considered for correcting low to moderate nearsightedness, farsightedness, or mild astigmatism, PRK is a surface ablation or photoablation procedure. The surgeon uses the excimer laser to ablate through the surface epithelium of the cornea and then reshape the corneal stroma surface. Unlike LASIK, no flap is cut on the surface of the cornea; instead, the surgeon uses the laser to reach the deeper corneal stromal tissue. Like LASIK, the procedure takes less than one minute per eye. A bandage contact lens is placed over the eyes after the operation and should be worn for three to seven days until the surface epithelium is healed.

Unfortunately, because of the surface ablation PRK generates significantly more discomfort and pain than LASIK. Also, the eye heals much more slowly: functional vision takes three to seven days with PRK, as opposed to one day for LASIK; complete healing takes three weeks to several months, as opposed to six weeks for LASIK. In addition, with PRK, you may experience corneal haze or a slight blurriness for a few weeks.

On the other hand, PRK is considered more versatile than LASIK. It can be performed on some people who should not have LASIK because their occupations or serious hobbies predispose them to eye trauma (for example, carpenters, construction workers, or tennis players), and dislodging the flap can cause serious complications. Furthermore, PRK can be performed on patients with thin, flat, or steep corneas, or other eye problems such as loosely adherent corneal epithelium, recurrent erosion syndrome, deep-seated eyes, or narrow fissures—patients who might not respond well to LASIK.

### LASEK (laser epithelial keratomileusis)

LASEK and epi-LASIK are two new techniques that have been developed in an attempt to combine the relative postoperative comfort of LASIK with the versatility of PRK. (Reports vary with regard to the relative success of these procedures.)

LASEK is technically a variation of PRK. In this procedure the surgeon covers the central cornea with an alcohol solution that loosens the edges of the epithelium. After the epithelium is loosened, the surgeon lifts the flap (consisting only of surface epithelium) with an instrument called a trephine and gently folds it back. The cornea is then treated with the excimer laser as it is with LASIK or PRK, and the epithelial flap is placed back over the eye. A bandage contact lens may be placed over the cornea to promote healing and comfort. The edges of the epithelium heal in four to seven days with recovery of functional vision, while stability of vision takes three weeks to several months. There is apt to be some pain for a few days.

### Epi-LASIK

In Epi-LASIK, as in LASIK, the surgeon creates a flap on the cornea, but the flap consists of only the epithelium, not the slightly deeper corneal tissue (the stroma). Instead of using alcohol to raise the epithelium as in LASEK, the surgeon uses an epikeratome and a suction ring to create pressure, then separates the epithelium as a sheet. The excimer laser is used to treat the cornea. A bandage contact lens is usually positioned at the end of the procedure. As in LASEK, the patient may experience some pain and blurry vision, which may last several days. The epithelium heals within a week for functional vision, and within a few months for full vision stability.

## FINDING A COMPETENT REFRACTIVE SURGEON

LASIK surgery is currently very popular, and also very commercial. Advertisements appear on television and radio, in magazines and newspapers, even on buses and subways. Although the doctors promoting these procedures may be excellent, I don't recommend choosing a surgeon from an advertisement. You wouldn't choose a heart surgeon or a cancer specialist that way—and of course the health of your eyes is every bit as important as that of any other part of your body.

The best referral to a LASIK surgeon is from your regular eye doctor. He may perform refractive surgery himself; if he does not, he will be able to advise you on the best places to go and the best surgeons to consult. If you do not have a regular

BOX 19

## Questions to Ask a Refractive Surgeon

I strongly recommend that you interview at least three refractive surgeons before you commit to having refractive surgery. In addition to the serious general questions you should ask about the procedure, if you have dry eye, you should clarify that the surgeon is aware of your special issues. You should ensure that he will pay attention to these issues before, during, and after the surgery. Here are some appropriate questions.

**1** *How many refractive procedures have you performed?*
The answer should be in the area of 500 procedures. (Remember, that figure may represent only 250 patients.)

**2** *How long have you been practicing refractive surgery?*
An experienced refractive surgeon should have been performing the procedure for at least three years.

**3** *What percent of your patients have reported problems or complications?*
The answer should certainly be less than 5 percent. Ask about the success rate among his patients. Probe about any who have had problems; ask how the problem was treated and how (or if) it was resolved.

**4** *What percentage of your patients ended up with 20/20 vision and are not experiencing distortion or aberration?*
One of the problems with refractive surgery is that the eye tests after surgery may indicate that patients are seeing extremely well, 20/20. However, they may be experiencing glare, haze, halos, and poor contrast, which makes vision not only less than perfect, but in some cases incapacitating. Discuss this issue with your doctor.

**5** *Because I have dry eye but still wish to have refractive surgery, what type of refractive surgery do you recommend?*
Most research today indicates that LASIK surgery results in the most frequent incidence of dry eye after refractive surgery. (Bear in mind, however, that dry eye symptoms are almost certain after all forms of refractive surgery, at least for the first few weeks.) Your doctor should discuss with you the various possibilities vis-à-vis the quality of your cornea (is it too thin for LASIK, for example?) and the nature of your dry eye problems.

**6** *What kind of presurgery evaluations do you perform on dry eye patients?*
If you have had dry eye for a long time, your doctor should be fully apprised not only of your dry eye problems, but of other health problems you may have (rheumatoid arthritis? diabetes?). He should evaluate for tear production, quality, and stability. Also, he should make sure that both aqueous tear deficient dry eye and meibomian gland disease have been under control for three months.

**7** *Do you see your patients postoperatively? Do you do your own follow-up?*
Many refractive surgeons have a high turnover of patients. They may have a comanagement practice. Make sure your surgeon will be available to you after the operation, especially if you suffer from dry eye.

**8** *Have you managed dry eye patients after refractive surgery?*
Don't be afraid to ask your doctor if he has treated other dry eye patients. He should indicate that he is very selective about recommending surgery to dry eye patients, and insists that all dry eye symptoms are under control and that the cornea is smooth and erosion free. He should also be open about dry eye therapies.

ophthalmologist or optometrist, check the American Academy of Ophthalmology website, or get in touch with refractive surgery offices in your area. Visit the offices and research the recommended surgeons carefully.

Because refractive surgery is a relatively new technique (and is changing rapidly), refractive surgeons have had varying levels of training. Some will have taken only the minimum course work necessary to be certified, while others have spent extra time (sometimes a year or two) performing refractive surgery as part of a special fellowship. Some may have been performing refractive surgery for years; others may have been doing it for only a few months. Interview at least three surgeons before you make a final decision, and don't be afraid to ask probing questions (see Box 19).

## PROBLEMS WITH REFRACTIVE SURGERY

Although statistics vary, more than 95 percent of people who elect to have LASIK (and other refractive surgeries, including PRK and LASEK) report satisfactory results. Most come away from the surgery with adequate long-distance vision, and while their vision may not be 20/20 in all cases, most say that their uncorrected vision is greatly improved.

Because refractive surgery instruments and procedures are constantly being improved, complications can often be resolved in various ways. Nevertheless, problems persist. One of the biggest complaints about refractive surgery is that people over age 40 still need eyeglasses for reading and other up-close work. Most individuals who have LASIK surgery do so in order to be free of glasses, so discovering that they still require reading glasses can be a huge disappointment. Other more serious problems with LASIK include:

Overcorrection
Undercorrection
Inflammation and infection

Double vision
Acute sensitivity to light
Glare, or halo or starburst effect
Difficulty driving at night, with perpetual glare and halos
Reduced contrast sensitivity (everything looks washed out)
Difficulty determining the power of intraocular lens replacement during potential future cataract surgery

These problems are usually relatively mild, but in a small percentage of cases they are severe and can have a significant negative effect on quality of life. This is especially true if dry eye develops or is exacerbated after refractive surgery.

## LASIK SURGERY AND DRY EYE

The relationship between LASIK surgery and dry eye is one of those chicken-and-egg situations so common when it comes to dry eye syndrome. LASIK surgery, for many reasons, often causes dry eye syndrome, especially immediately after the surgery and for a few months later, as the eyes heal. At the same time, many people who elect to have LASIK surgery do so because they already have dry eye—often owing to years of contact lens use. In fact, some can no longer tolerate wearing their contact lenses, which is why they choose to have the surgery. These people look to LASIK as a way to resolve their dry eye problems, freeing them from the bother of lenses, not to mention healing their painful, irritated eyes. Unfortunately, dry eye syndrome is often worse, not better, after LASIK.

### If You Have Dry Eye but Still Want Refractive Surgery

Some surgeons claim that even if you already have dry eye, you may still be able to have successful refractive surgery. However, it is imperative that your refractive surgeon and your general eye doctor be fully aware of your existing dry eye problems. Your eyes should be tested to determine tear quantity and quality.

Since LASIK surgery seems to be most commonly associated with dry eye (because of the disruption of corneal nerves), your doctor(s) may suggest that you consider PRK, LASEK, or epi-LASIK instead. Make no mistake, though, all of these procedures will affect your corneal sensation and tear function to some extent.

Again, do your homework. For example, studies suggest that certain types of LASIK flaps may reduce dry eye symptoms somewhat. Specifically, a wider flap with its hinge on the nasal side of the cornea rather than on top has been found, in some cases, to preserve better corneal sensation leading to better tear function. You might want to question your surgeon about these findings or others you come across in your research.

In any case, it is imperative that the ocular surface be healthy before refractive surgery. If dry eye has been a problem, the symptoms must be brought under control and the surface of the cornea must be smooth without erosions before the operation to ensure the best results.

## Post-LASIK Dry Eye

According to some statistics, at least 60 percent of LASIK patients have problems with dry eye—at least to some degree—in the first month after LASIK surgery. Although for most post-LASIK patients dry eye subsides as the eyes heal and is usually resolved after six months, for many it does not. In some cases the dry eye gets worse.

After LASIK surgery, dry eye may develop for many reasons. Because the cornea has been desensitized through the cutting of nerves in the corneal surface, the signals for the lacrimal gland to secrete watery tears are not triggered, so fewer tears appear. Signals for lipid production and secretion in the meibomian glands and the normal blink may also be affected. Because of the suction pressure applied during LASIK, the goblet cells in the conjunctiva may become damaged and the mucin production interrupted; as a result, the tear film becomes unstable. Finally, because the curvature of the cornea has been flattened, and a

BOX 20

**Warning!**

If you suspect you are suffering from dry eye after having had LASIK surgery, it is crucial that you see your doctor immediately. Don't try to self-treat with over-the-counter products. Not only will you continue to experience pain and discomfort, but severe inflammation or infection may develop, which could jeopardize your eyes and your vision. Again, if you are experiencing pain or other dry eye symptoms, see your doctor right away!

space (or spaces) may have been created between the lid and the cornea, the eyelid may not glide properly over the cornea, thus affecting tear distribution over the surface.

In other words, the entire tear-producing mechanism can be affected by LASIK. The result may be aqueous tear deficient dry eye, evaporative dry eye, or both. Chronic inflammation may ensue, with further loss of tear function. Even worse, if eyedrops are prescribed, you may be allergic to them.

Post-LASIK dry eye is treated precisely the same way as any other case of dry eye. Your doctor may prescribe liquid tears (without preservatives) and a lubricating ointment, as well as a mild steroid (Lotemax) or cyclosporin (Restasis) to deal with any inflammation. Some patients may benefit from an autologous serum, obtained by drawing their blood, separating out the serum, and combining it with a saline solution, thereby creating a very effective eyedrop for dry eye. A punctal occlusion may be required to be sure your eyes are getting sufficient tears. If meibomian gland disease is present, you may need oral doxycycline (an antibiotic). Some patients benefit from nutritional supplements, while others find relief via amniotic membrane or other eye surgery designed to stabilize the ocular surface.

## FINAL THOUGHTS

In the course of my practice, I have treated many patients suffering from eye problems that were a direct result of LASIK and other refractive surgeries. Although these surgeries are miraculous in many ways—and most people who have LASIK surgery are extremely pleased with the results—because of the huge numbers of people having the surgery, the small percentage of problem cases is actually a significant number of people. Their problems may not be easily detected or documented, given the limits of today's diagnostic vision tests. A patient may indeed have 20/20 vision after LASIK, but still may suffer from glare, halos, double vision, and other problems that profoundly affect vision but don't necessarily show up when the patient is tested.

With regard to dry eye, although I have been able to relieve most of the subjective post-LASIK dry eye pain of my patients, I have been concerned about the number of individuals whose symptoms in those rare, severe cases may be debilitating, if not incapacitating. Bear in mind that refractive surgery is absolute; it cannot be undone. It is imperative that you choose an excellent doctor for your surgery, and that you discuss any and all related medical problems—specifically including any history of dry eye—with the doctor beforehand.

Refractive surgery can bring wonderful relief. The technology is always improving; as a result, the surgery is becoming more exact and less risky. But for the time being, I strongly recommend that you approach refractive surgery with care and knowledge, especially if you have dry eye.

CHAPTER

# 9

# The Diagnosis

Myth

*Dry eye may not have any detectable abnormality to explain the symptoms.*

Fact

*Virtually all symptoms of dry eye can be traced to abnormalities of the lids and/or surface of the eye—even if the abnormalities are not initially apparent.*

Dry eye syndrome is an extremely complex malady. However, if you are a dry eye sufferer, most likely the one fact that is totally clear to you is your pain! And no doubt that extreme eye pain is what has driven you to see your doctor—and to read this book.

For doctors, the difficulty in diagnosing and treating dry eye syndrome is its very complexity. The cause of your pain—and the appropriate treatment for your pain—can be hard to pinpoint. Therefore, it is an enormous help to your doctor if you are as knowledgeable as you can be about dry eye syndrome in general and about your own overall health history, including your eye pain.

My goal in this chapter is to give you as much ammunition as possible to help your doctor find the cause of your dry eye, and to fight it effectively.

## FINDING THE RIGHT DOCTOR

The first step in treating your dry eye pain is to find and work with an appropriate eye doctor. This is imperative. You may have gone to the same eye doctor for years or, conversely, you may have *never* gone to an eye doctor. Indeed, many people have been fitted for glasses to treat their everyday refraction problems (nearsightedness, farsightedness, and the like) or their general eye problems by an optometrist and have never felt the need to see a medical eye doctor, that is, an ophthalmologist. Only when they begin to have serious health problems—such as acute eye pain—do they realize that perhaps they should see a medical doctor.

As it turns out, many are confused by the names given to the various eye care professionals: ophthalmologist, optometrist, and optician. It is important to know what each type of professional does, as well as why and when you may need him. (For the sake of simplicity, in this book I refer to eye care professionals using male pronouns, but of course many first-rate ophthalmologists, optometrists, and opticians are women.

### The Various Eye Professionals

An *ophthalmologist* is a medical doctor who specializes in care of the eyes. His training is normally quite extensive. He has a four-year undergraduate degree from a college or university; a four-year degree from an accredited medical school; one year of internship and three years of residency in ophthalmology (the study and care of the eyes); and very often, a postgraduate fellowship (usually one to three years) in some specific aspect of ophthalmology, such as glaucoma, the retina, cataracts, pediatric ophthalmology, neuro-ophthalmology, refractive surgery, or the cornea, and other external diseases including dry eye.

An ophthalmologist conducts examinations to determine the quality of vision and the need for corrective glasses. More than that, he checks for the presence of all eye diseases or disorders, including cataracts, glaucoma, macular degeneration, detached retina, and dry eye. As a trained physician, the ophthalmologist diagnoses not just eye diseases but also systemic diseases and other medical problems. He can prescribe medication and perform eye surgery, as necessary. An ophthalmologist may also prescribe glasses and contact lenses.

An *optometrist* is a health care professional trained to assess, by testing, the quality of vision; establish whether glasses or contact lenses are needed to improve vision; and prescribe appropriate glasses or contact lenses (optometry). An optometrist has completed a preprofessional undergraduate education at a college or university, plus four years of professional education at a college of optometry to earn a doctor of optometry (O.D.) degree. Some optometrists also have an optional residency in a special area of optometry. Although an optometrist may diagnose, treat, and manage certain diseases, injuries, and disorders of the eye, he is not a medical doctor and therefore may not prescribe all types of drugs or perform various surgeries. At the same time, many optometrists are able to diagnose ophthalmic or systemic problems, such as the onset of glaucoma, cataracts, or other diseases. Often an optometrist will refer patients who require advanced medical or surgical care to an ophthalmologist.

An *optician* is a person who practices opticianry, the filling of prescriptions for glasses and contact lenses. An optician may fit or adjust glasses, but is not certified to test eyes or prescribe glasses or contact lenses. Sometimes an optician is also an optometrist, or has a professional optometrist associated with his office or shop to test and prescribe glasses and contacts. Conversely, an optician may operate an optical shop that is part of the larger office of an ophthalmologist or optometrist.

If you are suffering from dry eye and are not responding to a routine regimen of artificial tears, you should consult with your optometrist or ophthalmologist. If your case is difficult to manage or severe, you may have serious medical problems. Therefore, you may want to be checked by an ophthalmologist. Specifically, look for an ophthalmologist who has special training (postresidency fellowship training) in the cornea, the ocular surface, or dry eye syndrome.

Finding a new doctor is as much a subjective task as it is an objective one. Objectively, you will want to know your doctor's educational background, amount and type of postgraduate training, level of experience (that is, how many years he has been practicing), and specifically if he has had experience treating dry eye. However, you must also trust your more subjective instincts when deciding if a doctor of any kind is right for you. This caveat applies as much to eye doctors as it does to gynecologists or cancer surgeons. When dealing with a syndrome as elusive as dry eye, the need for a doctor whom you are comfortable with and trust is even more important.

Whether you have been seeing the same eye doctor for decades or are in the process of finding a new one, consider these questions carefully:

Does my doctor spend enough time with me? Or does he rush me in and out of his office and routinely keep me waiting for long periods?

Does he make me feel comfortable? Does he show respect for me? Or do I sense that he is annoyed or impatient with me or my questions?

Does he really listen to my comments and questions?

Does he ask me questions in return? (Questions from the doctor indicate not only that he is listening, but that he is considering all possible ramifications of the problems.)

Does my doctor give answers that I understand? If I don't understand something, does he give clear, compassionate explanations?

Do I trust that he is doing everything he can to deal with my dry eye problems?

BOX 21

**Finding a Great Eye Doctor**

The following are excellent sources for finding an appropriate eye doctor.

Family members and friends. These are perhaps the best resources for doctors of any kind. A close friend or family member will give a straightforward assessment and will be concerned primarily with your welfare.

Your primary care physician. Your PCP is usually a valuable source for references to other doctors; however, recognize that he may recommend friends or close colleagues.

Your local hospital. Call the public relations office of a local hospital and ask for recommendations; realize, however, that the public relations person likely will only give you names of eye doctors who are staff members.

Your insurance company or health plan. Most insurance companies provide listings of doctors who honor their plans, so consult the carrier's catalogue or make contact by telephone or email. (Bear in mind that the recommended doctors are merely professionals who honor your health plan; the listings do not reflect competence.)

American Academy of Ophthalmology. This is a large national professional association, and most certified ophthalmologists are members. The AAO provides online listings (*www.aao.org*) of member ophthalmologists practicing in the United States and abroad, and includes each doctor's specialty, location, and telephone number. You can search by region or by specialty.

State ophthalmologic societies. Through the AAO, you can get a complete listing of all fifty state ophthalmologic societies and associations, together with the name of each director, an email address, and a website.

American Board of Medical Specialties Compendium. This listing gives all board-certified ophthalmologists in the United States, together with some biographical information, but does not rate doctors. Find it at your local library, call 866-ASK-ABMS (275-2267), or go online to *www.abms.org/member.asp.*

American Optometric Association. Your state optometric association can provide you with information about doctors of optometry in your area. To obtain the number of the association in your state, go to the AOA website: *www.aoa.org.*

Seniors Eyecare Program. This program provides referrals for U.S. citizens or legal residents, aged 65 or older, who do not have access to an ophthalmologist. Eligible callers are mailed the name of a volunteer ophthalmologist in their community. For seniors without the means to pay, the exam and treatment are free. Call 1.800.222.EYES, or go to the Seniors Eyecare website: *www.eyecareamerica.org.*

After weighing these matters, if you discover that you are in any way uncomfortable or displeased with your doctor, look for someone else. Even if you have gone to the same doctor for years or if your new doctor comes highly recommended and has impeccable credentials, if you are not fully confident that you can work with him, don't hesitate to seek another doctor. Box 21 gives you some suggestions about how to look.

## THE EYE EXAM AHEAD

### Preparing Ahead

Regardless of whether you are visiting a doctor you have known for decades or are meeting a new eye doctor for the first time, you need to take time to create a report not only about your dry eye problems, but about your health in general. (See Box 22.) Your doctor will probably not ask you many of these questions, but come prepared with your answers anyway, and consider them carefully. Be sure to give him all your information, even if he doesn't ask for it.

### Simple Questions Yield Complex Results

At least half a dozen professional dry eye questionnaires are available, including McMonnies Dry Eye Index, the Impact of Dry Eye on Everyday Life (IDEEL), and Dry Eye Questionnaire 2001 (DEQ). One of the most popular among doctors is a well-respected professional questionnaire called the Ocular Surface Disease Index, which can be accessed on the Internet at *www.dryeyeeducation.com/OSDI.pdf.* Your doctor may ask you to take this test or one like it, but you might want to "test" yourself before you go for your appointment. The questions can help you pinpoint your symptoms, and by analyzing your answers, you'll have a clear idea of the seriousness of your dry eye problems.

### The Doctor-Patient Interview

When you arrive at the doctor's office for your eye examination, be prepared to spend about an hour. (Bear in mind that this is an estimate, since each doctor is different.) In my office, an office assistant fills out the paperwork, which takes about fifteen minutes, then an ophthalmic technician obtains a baseline general history, including checking your visual acuity on the eye chart and the accuracy of the prescription for your glasses. I usually

BOX 22

**Your Dry Eye History: A Checklist**

Bring the following information with you when you visit your ophthalmologist:

**1** *A list of your dry eye symptoms and the length of time you have experienced them.*
Very likely, you can quickly and easily list your specific dry eye symptoms. But to ensure that you include them all, reread the section on symptoms in Chapter 1. And take the Ocular Surface Disease Index OSDI© test, found at *www.dryeyeeducation.com/OSDI.pdf.*

**2** *Comments on the following factors:*
When do your symptoms occur? (Upon awakening? Late in the day? The middle of the night?)
What aggravates your symptoms? (Reading? Watching TV? Working on the computer? Driving? Sleeping? Fragrances or perfumes?)
What relieves your symptoms? (Blinking? Eyedrops? Squinting? Closing your eyes?)

**3** *A history of your contact lens wear, if any.*
(How long have you worn them? Do you wear rigid lenses? Soft lenses? Extended-wear lenses? When did you first notice problems with your lenses?)

**4** *For women, your status with regard to menopause, including* hormone replacement therapy—type, dosage, and length of time you have been taking the drug.

**5** *A list of all medications you are currently taking, including:*

Prescription medications, including dosage

Nonprescription medications, including aspirin and over-the-counter eyedrops

Vitamins and herbal supplements

Any allergies to medications

**6** *Information about any eye diseases, injuries, or surgeries you have had at any time in your life, including:*

Any serious eye disease (cataracts, glaucoma, macular degeneration, retinal detachment, and so on)

Any serious eye injury

Chronic allergies that have affected your eyes

Any other disease or disorder that has affected your eyes in any way

**7** *A family history of any serious or chronic eye problem* (especially parents, siblings, or children), even if you have not been diagnosed with it yourself.

**8** *Information about any serious or chronic non–eye-related health problems and surgeries you may have, including:*

Chronic asthma or other allergies

Skin conditions (psoriasis, eczema, seborrhea, rosacea)

Nose and throat problems

A multiorgan disease, such as diabetes, lupus, or rheumatoid arthritis

Sleep problems

Psychiatric problems, including medications such as antidepressants, antipsychotics, medication for bipolar disorder

Neurologic diseases, including stroke, Parkinson's disease

Gastrointestinal diseases

Kidney diseases

**9** *Information about personal everyday activities that might possibly affect your dry eye. For example:*

Do you smoke? How much?

Do you drink more than two alcoholic beverages every day? Have you been treated for alcoholism or any other drug-related problem?

During the day do you drink more than two cups of coffee, tea, or other caffeinated beverage such as soda?

Do you consume an excessive amount of chocolate on a daily basis?

Do you eat foods containing high levels of omega-3 fatty acids such as tuna, salmon, sardines, mackerel, herring, or lake trout several times every week?

Do you work and/or live in an exceptionally dry environment?

Do you work and/or live in an exceptionally cool environment?

Do you regularly engage in any sports (bicycling; driving; skiing) that may dry out your eyes?

Do you use fans of any sort, including ceiling, floor, and desk fans?

Do you have pets or regularly come in contact with animals?

spend between thirty and ninety minutes with each new patient, depending on the complexity of the problems, to perform a comprehensive examination.

The doctor will probably ask for your summary of the symptoms you are experiencing, which may include some or all of the classic dry eye symptoms: pain, grittiness, scratchiness, foreign object, burning, and itching. However, he may also inquire about other health issues seemingly unrelated to dry eye. What's more, these topics may seem quite personal.

For example, your doctor may ask about aspects of your sex life: your form of birth control and birth control pills, pregnancies, lactation, menopause, hormone replacement, surgery or diseases involving the sex organs (ovaries and testes as well as the adrenal gland), and other questions touching on sexuality and personal relationships. We have seen that the sex hormones, particularly androgen and estrogen, can have much to do with causing dry eye, and it is imperative that you answer all of these questions fully to help the doctor diagnose and properly treat your eye problems.

Be as open, honest, and informative as possible. Don't hesitate to ask your eye doctor to clarify any of his comments that you don't completely understand. Be especially sure that you are clear about how to take any medications he prescribes. If you are worried about understanding what the doctor says, or if you have trouble hearing, bring a relative or friend with you to your appointment. You may want to ask that person to write down the doctor's instructions.

## Noneye Considerations

Before the doctor even looks at your eyes, he'll examine a host of other physical aspects that may relate to your eyes—and to your dry eye. Although he will probably not perform a complete physical, he will look at a range of physical problems that can relate to dry eye in one way or another.

- Head and neck. Your doctor may feel the sides and back of your head, the base of your skull, and your neck. Pain in this area, called occipital tenderness, is usually caused by tense muscles at the base of the skull and neck, which may be experienced as pain in the eyes.
- Lymph nodes. If the lymph nodes in front of the ears or under the jawbone on the side of the neck are swollen, a viral infection may be indicated.

- Sinuses. If your sinuses are tender, you may simply have a cold or possibly a bacterial infection. However, if you are taking antihistamines as therapy to treat the cold, the medication may be exacerbating your dry eye symptoms.
- Facial scars. Scars from burns or other traumas as well as from shingles or chronic acne may be present on your forehead or face. Your doctor will be quick to conclude that the burn, trauma, or shingles may have affected the surface of the eye or the tear glands. Scars from acne indicate problems with sebaceous glands, which may point to meibomian gland dysfunction.
- Rosacea. With rosacea, red dilated blood vessels and blotchiness are usually evident on your face and indicate that the sebaceous glands there are inflamed. If your eyelids are also irritated, it means that your meibomian glands are affected, implying possible meibomian gland dysfunction. Rosacea sufferers tend to have decreased tear clearance, because the inflammatory nature of the disease reduces the outflow of tears through swollen tear drainage ducts. As a result, microbes, irritants, and other materials are not flushed out of the eyes, which can lead to inflammation from allergies, toxicities, and ultimately an extremely irritated and dry eye.
- Eczema. Signs of eczema anywhere on the body suggest an atopic allergic disease, such as asthma or hay fever. Being atopic places the patient at risk for a range of eye problems from conjunctivitis (with vision-threatening scarring) to blepharitis, cataracts, retinal detachment, and herpes simplex infections.
- Arthritis in your hands. Signs of arthritis, particularly in your hands, may indicate Sjögren's syndrome (rheumatoid arthritis). Also, they may alert your doctor to potential trouble administering your eyedrops and other medications.
- Hemorrhages under the nails. Hemorrhages in the shape of splinters under the finger (or toe) nails may indicate

undiagnosed lupus or other serious systemic disease, which may ultimately affect the eyes.

- Dry mouth with little saliva suggests possible Sjögren's syndrome.

As you can see, while your doctor is ostensibly checking you in order to treat your dry eye, he may also find as yet undiagnosed problems (lupus, for example), or see issues that need to be taken into account when deciding on treatment.

## Examining the Eyes and Eyelids

After taking a look at your upper body, including your face, head, neck, and hands, the doctor will conduct a comprehensive examination of your eyes. He will start by checking whether your eyes move normally, whether your pupils are dilating and constricting properly, and whether your peripheral vision is appropriate. He will then check your eyelids, starting with your blink rate and whether the upper and lower lids touch with each blink. This will be followed by an examination of how well the eyelid closes over the eye, specifically looking for incomplete eyelid closure, or lagophthalmos. The doctor will look for any excessive squinting or pulling of the outer corners of the eyelid. Finally, he will check for other diseases and disorders that can affect the eyelids and that may directly or indirectly cause dry eye: proper eyelid-eyeball apposition, lashes rubbing against the cornea (trichiasis), droopy eyelids (ptosis), discharge of the eyelid margins (blepharitis or infection), and floppy lids.

## Inspecting for Dry Eye

Having looked into these other aspects, the doctor will check for signs to explain your dry eye symptoms. Initially, he'll look at the most overt and obvious signals: redness and inflammation, squinting, and anything else he can see without the help of special equipment or tests.

BOX 23

**Case Study: Laura**

Laura was a 24-year-old college student with a history of juvenile rheumatoid arthritis, as well as chronic inflammation of the left eye that was being treated by a variety of doctors. Her condition left her with decreased vision from an opaque cornea, and she was sent to me for a cornea transplant. I performed the transplant and her sight improved. After a few weeks she developed significant, excruciating pain in her eye. No abnormality appeared to account for her terrible eye pain; however, the pain soon became so intolerable that she told her other doctors that she wanted to have the eye removed—clearly an extreme solution.

Before the planned surgery, she returned to me for an appointment to follow up on her transplant. I observed that the muscles at the base of her skull were extremely tight (she had been under a lot of stress) and wondered if they were also squeezing the nerves buried within the muscles, causing not only localized neck pain but also referred pain in her eye. To test my hypothesis, I injected a local anesthetic into the muscles in her neck. Laura experienced immediate relief not only in her neck, but in her eye as well. Within minutes her pain had almost vanished. She was not only amazed that her pain had disappeared so quickly, but was shaken by the realization that she could have sacrificed her eye needlessly. She was treated over the long term with massage therapy, heat, and muscle relaxants, which kept her pain in check.

Your doctor may turn to a few pieces of traditional equipment to help make his diagnosis. These may include:

- A slitlamp biomicroscope. Known commonly as a slitlamp, this instrument consists of a microscope combined with a light source and is used to examine the entire eye from front to back, including the tear film, cornea, aqueous humor, lens, vitreous, retina, and optic nerve. The slitlamp helps detect anatomical problems that may be contributing to dry eye symptoms. For example, the lacrimal gland can be examined to make sure that that it is not enlarged or its ducts scarred shut, or the meibomian gland can be checked for plugging.
- A transilluminator. This device permits light to shine through the eyelid, revealing the meibomian glands. If the glands are blocked or atrophied, the problems will be evident.
- A filter. This is a hand-held device with a yellow filter that enhances fluorescein stain, increasing the doctor's ability to locate subtle problems with the surface of the eye.

In order to diagnose dry eye in all its facets, your doctor may also perform a number of traditional tests commonly used to assess tear quantity and quality as well as to check the state of the cornea and the conjunctiva. These tests include:

- Schirmer test. This test is used to assess aqueous tear production, or the amount of tears a patient is producing. Tiny filter paper strips are folded over the lower lid margin and removed after five minutes. When the strips are removed, the dampened area is measured in millimeters.

  I sometimes perform serial Schirmer tests, one immediately after the other. Sometimes aqueous tear production can initially appear to be satisfactory, but upon a second or third test may prove to be inadequate.

  A Schirmer test can be performed with or without anesthetic. I usually use an anesthetic in the form of a drop;

it eliminates reflex tearing, which can skew the test and make it difficult to pick up certain cases of dryness.

- Fluorescein/TBUT test. This test, used to evaluate the tear breakup time (TBUT) to give an indication of tear stability, is performed by applying fluorescein dye to the tear film. The patient is asked to blink several times to distribute the fluorescein, then to not blink. The time is measured until the tear film begins to break up, with dry spots appearing on the corneal surface.

  The tear breakup time is decreased in patients with dry eye (the normal TBUT is at least ten seconds). With an abnormal test, secretions of mucin from the goblet cells or lipid secretion from meibomian glands may be the cause, although TBUT can also indicate problems with aqueous tears. The pattern of breakup may suggest one type of tear deficiency rather than another.
- Rose bengal staining and lissamine green test. These "color" tests are used to assess the health of the conjunctiva epithelial cells. The rose bengal will check that the cells are adequately coated with mucin, while the lissamine green will reveal cells undergoing degeneration.
- Tear clearance test. By analyzing the ability of the eye to clear a precise amount of fluorescein dye from its surface, this test judges "tear turnover," or how effectively the eye removes old tears and is replenished with new tears. It also indicates abnormal aqueous tear production and meibomian gland dysfunction.
- MRIs and other special tests. For various reasons, your doctor may decide to perform certain other tests, normally done out of the office. These may include laboratory blood tests to check for Sjögren's syndrome, lupus, diabetes, or other diseases. He may decide to order a CT (computerized topography) scan or an MRI (magnetic resonance imaging) scan if he suspects a less common cause for dry eye such as a tumor in the lacrimal system or Graves' disease. Ordering special out-of-office tests is infrequent, however.

BOX 24

**Case Study: Matthew**

Matthew was a 45-year-old electrician who was suffering from many symptoms of dry eye, especially scratchiness and a grainy sensation in the eyes that he experienced throughout the day. Convinced he had dry eye, he had gone to two or three doctors who had run standard tests, including a Schirmer test, and found that his eyes were normal. Still, Matthew experienced severe eye pain. Over-the-counter drops gave him no relief and he remained convinced he had dry eye.

Finally, a friend recommended that he come to see me. After listening to his story, I decided to try giving him two serial Schirmer tests instead of the conventional single test. Also, I opted to test one eye at a time to minimize reflex tearing. The results showed significant lack of tear production in Matthew's eyes. It appeared that his aqueous tear secretion was inadequate, a result that sometimes does not show up with a single Schirmer test. I cauterized his tear drainage canal (punctal occlusion) and suggested that he use preservative-free artificial tears for sensitive eyes. Today he is pain free.

## THE DOCTOR'S DIAGNOSIS

It is not usually necessary for a doctor to perform an extensive battery of tests in order to make an accurate diagnosis. The approach I use is to simplify the complexity of the symptoms by first identifying the various ocular surface abnormalities. These abnormalities are prioritized for treatment, according to which conditions account for the majority of symptoms. The conditions are then targeted with specific therapy. Since no two patients are the same, obviously each patient's treatment must be individualized.

For example, if a patient's Schirmer test score is high (meaning his aqueous tear secretion is adequate), but his TBUT is low (indicating that the tear film is breaking up quickly and the film is destabilized), I would expect to treat problems with the meibomian glands and lipid tear or the goblet cells and mucin production, or an irregular corneal surface. If both the Schirmer test and the TBUT are low (indicating problems with at least the aqueous tear secretion), I would first initiate therapy addressing the aqueous tear deficiency. Of course, I would also look for other surface problems such as allergy and blepharitis and treat them accordingly.

Diagnosis and treatment of dry eye depend on an accurate and comprehensive understanding of the disease in general and of your symptoms in particular. Because dry eye disease is so complex and results from such a broad range of causes, the more facts you provide your eye doctor to help him diagnose your problem, the more quickly you will find relief.

CHAPTER

# 10

# Treatment

Myth

*All cases of dry eye can be easily treated with over-the-counter eyedrops.*

Fact

*Dry eye, especially when it becomes severe, is an extremely complex disorder, and the necessary treatment is as multifaceted as the cause.*

As we've seen repeatedly, dry eye syndrome is extremely complicated and can be caused by any number of variables from prolonged contact lens wear to a severe case of Sjögren's syndrome. For doctors, it may be difficult to diagnose properly, and it may be difficult to treat.

## LEVELS OF SEVERITY AND LEVELS OF TREATMENT

In April 2004 an international panel of doctors and researchers presented its recommendations for the treatment of dry eye disease, using the Delphi Consensus Approach. (The name refers to a concept that goes back to the ancient Greek oracle of Delphi, who offered wisdom and advice from the "elders" or "sages." Today the Delphi Consensus Approach is a scientific method of assembling a consensus of information from experts on a particular subject, here the definition and treatment of dry eye disease.) This distinguished panel of doctors from around the world concluded that "severity of the disease" was the most important factor in the choice of treatment for dry eye syndrome.

The Delphi panel defined four levels of severity, based on symptoms and signs. ("Symptoms" are subjective irritations and pains experienced by the patient, whereas "signs" are objective test results or clinical observations made by the doctor.) The four levels are 1, Mild; 2, Moderate; 3, Severe; and 4, Extremely Severe. After defining the levels of severity, the panel assigned recommended treatments for each level with or without lid margin disease (see Box 25).

My own initial approach to therapy is similar to that recommended by the Delphi panel. However, because no two patients are identical, my final chosen therapy (as with most physicians, of course) reflects the needs of the specific patient being evaluated.

## When to See Your Doctor

Even if your dry eye symptoms are only somewhat painful or irritating and you believe you have only a mild case, I strongly recommend that you see your eye doctor for a baseline checkup when you suspect that you have dry eye, or indeed any chronic problem with your eyes. (A "chronic problem" would be pain or irritation for, say, two weeks without relief from over-the-counter eyedrops. Obviously, with any significant acute or sudden pain or change in vision, you should be seen by your eye doctor immediately.)

Dry eye syndrome can be caused by any number of factors, including a serious systemic disease. In addition, since chronic dry eye paradoxically can lead to reduced ocular sensation, you may actually have an advanced case of dry eye but experience only mild symptoms. If your doctor finds that you are suffering only from "mild" dry eye, then basic remedies should be sufficient. However, he may discover that your dry eye is more serious than you suspected, and he will probably begin a more rigorous treatment immediately.

BOX 25

## Delphi Dry Eye Treatment Recommendations

Note: This chart, based on the Delphi consensus, appeared in marginally different form in the July 15, 2005, issue of *Ophthalmology Times,* as well as in several other professional publications. I have revised it slightly and have added to the treatment recommendations for Level 1 and Level 2.

### Level 1. Mild Dry Eye

Signs and Symptoms

Mild to moderate symptoms
Mild to moderate conjunctival signs; no corneal signs

Treatment Recommendations

Patient (and family) counseling and education
Eliminate (minimize) environmental factors
Eliminate (minimize) drug factors
Identify and control allergies
Minimize enabling personal habits
Consider dietary issues
Over-the-counter preserved tears

If no improvement, add Level 2 treatment

### Level 2. Moderate Dry Eye

Signs and Symptoms

Moderate to severe symptoms
Signs of tear film instability
Mild corneal punctate staining
Conjunctival staining
Visible inflammation

Treatment Recommendations

"Transient" (nonpreserved) tears over-the-counter
Gels/ointments
Cyclosporin A
Topical steroids
Secretagogues
Punctal plugs and cautery (after inflammation is controlled)

If no improvement, add Level 3 treatment

**Level 3. Severe Dry Eye**

Signs and Symptoms

Severe symptoms
Marked corneal punctate staining
Central corneal staining
Filamentary keratitis

Treatment Recommendations

Oral tetracyclines
Autologous serum

If no improvement, add Level 4 treatment

**Level 4. Extremely Severe Dry Eye**

Signs and Symptoms

Severe symptoms
Severe corneal staining
Conjunctival scarring

Treatment Recommendations

Systemic anti-inflammatory therapy
Topical vitamin-A therapy
Acetylcysteine
Moisture goggles
Surgery

For starters, he will give you a brief overview of what is involved with dry eye treatment and he will perform various tests (Schirmer, dye staining, tear breakup time) in order to define the severity of your problem. He will probably give you guidelines (see Box 25) regarding the various therapies, from over-the-counter medications to surgery. Most therapy will involve keeping the eyes lubricated and reducing inflammation.

## TREATING LEVEL 1 DRY EYE

Mild dry eye is characterized by classic mild to moderate dry eye symptoms, including scratchiness, grittiness, graininess, a burning sensation, or a foreign body sensation. These symptoms may be intermittent, occurring as a result of certain stressful eye conditions (such as long hours working at a computer or behind the wheel of a car), or they may be constant.

While annoying and probably painful at times, mild dry eye is not vision threatening. If you have mild aqueous tear deficient dry eye, you may need to begin a simple regimen of over-the-counter artificial tears as well as take a few additional precautions. If you show signs of meibomian gland dysfunction, blepharitis, allergies, sinusitis, or other related problems, you'll need to treat these disorders as well.

### Counseling and Education

Certain basic factors should be taken into account before you begin medical treatment for your dry eye—even if you will just be putting over-the-counter drops in your eyes.

As a dry eye sufferer, you need to understand your disease; in other words, you require some information and education. Reading magazine and newspaper articles, carefully checking out books such as this one, and consulting various websites on the subject are advisable.

You should also take care of some basic factors regarding your general health. These include making sure you are eating a balanced diet, staying well hydrated, practicing appropriate personal hygiene, getting adequate sleep, and exercising regularly, all of which will contribute to keeping dry eye in check. Protect your eyes while outdoors from the sun and wind with wraparound sunglasses. Make sure that any other medical conditions you may have, such as diabetes or severe allergies, are under control.

Close family members should know you have dry eye so that they can help you cope. They can identify personal habits you may not be aware of that are detrimental to your dry eye, such as constantly rubbing your eyes. They can help maintain a home environment friendly to dry eye by keeping air humidified, not smoking, and turning off ceiling fans when you are in the room. They can remind you to use your therapy and inform you if your eyes are looking red and irritated.

### Consider Your Environment

The moment you suspect you might have dry eye syndrome, you need to take a close look at your environment. This includes not just the general geographical region where you live, but your specific household surroundings, your work atmosphere (especially your use of a computer), your recreational life, even the environmental conditions in your automobile, particularly if you spend hours behind the wheel. (See Chapter 11 for a number of practical suggestions.) Precautions with regard to all facets of your personal environment are as important as medical solutions in the treatment of dry eye disease.

### Take Stock of All Medications

Make a detailed list of all medications you are taking for any disease or disorder, from the common cold to more serious disorders such as depression, menopausal problems, Parkinson's disease, high blood pressure, diabetes, or Sjögren's syndrome. Include all over-the-counter medications, especially cold and allergy remedies (they usually contain antihistamines, which exacerbate dry eye), herbal remedies, and, of course, all prescription medications for additional current or chronic disorders including allergies and depression. Be sure to note any allergies you may have to over-the-counter or prescription medications.

In consultation with your doctor, you may be able to minimize or eliminate the drying effect on the eye from some of your medications by reducing the dosage, changing a medication to a nondrying type, or discontinuing it altogether. *Warning:* Do not make decisions about changing medications, especially prescription medications, without consulting your physician.

### Check Your Allergies

If you have allergies, your doctor needs to work closely with you so that you are treating both your allergies and your dry eye effectively. As we have seen, certain allergies can cause or exacerbate dry eye, and certain allergy medications may be problematic with regard to dry eye. Allergy-related problems, particularly sinusitis (inflamed or infected sinuses), can cause decreased tear clearance and inflammation and lead to dry eye symptoms.

Be sure to inform your doctor of any allergies you may have and, again, give him a complete rundown of all medications, prescription or over the counter, that you use to treat those allergies. (You may be asked to see an allergist for skin testing to identify specific allergies you may have.)

### Minimize Problematic Personal Habits

Many people who suffer from even mild dry eye develop habits such as chronically rubbing their eyes, constantly wiping their eyes rather than blotting them with tissues, or using their fingers to remove mucus or other debris that can collect in the eyes. These habits need to be identified and eliminated.

Some people use (and reuse!) handkerchiefs—or even paper

tissues—to perform double duty for the nose and the eyes. This habit can bring all sorts of microorganisms to the eye, which can cause irritation and possibly infection. Use a clean tissue whenever you dab your eyes. Wash your hands regularly to reduce the presence of potential allergens and microbes from your fingers; better yet, try to avoid touching the eyes with your fingers at all. Instead, when your eyes are irritated, rinse them with over-the-counter sterile eye rinse and blot them dry with a clean tissue.

## Dietary Issues

### *Omega-3 Fatty Acids*

The role of essential omega-3 fatty acids is one of the hottest topics of the day in dry eye treatment, since it has been found anecdotally that increasing these fatty acids in the diet stimulates healthy lipid and aqueous tear production. Omega-3 fatty acids are found in wild (as opposed to farm-raised) fish, especially tuna, salmon, mackerel, and sardines, as well as in fish oil. One study found that adding tuna fish (at least five servings per week) to the diet was effective in reducing the rate of dry eye in women.

Omega-3 fatty acids are also found in flaxseed oil. Several years ago, Carl F. Boerner, a Boston-based ophthalmologist, presented data she had gleaned from her practice, where she studied the effect of flaxseed oil on dry eye patients. She found that flaxseed oil relieved the symptoms in 85 percent of her patients. (Later, flaxseed oil was also found to help increase contact lens wearing time in patients with borderline dry eyes and contact lens intolerance.) Flaxseed oil is one of the world's richest sources of omega-3 fatty acids; in fact, it contains twice as much as fish oil. Specifically, flaxseed oil contains alpha-linolenic acid omega-3 (57 percent); linolenic acid omega-6 (15 percent); and oleic acid omega-9 (18 percent). Flaxseed oil can be purchased in health food stores in seed, capsule, or liquid form.

### *Other Nutritional Considerations*

In recent years, experts have found that nutrition is an increasingly important factor in treating dry eye. The following are among the most interesting findings.

*Water Intake.* Experts have found that simply by increasing the amount of water you consume every day, dry eye symptoms may be controlled. A healthy diet includes about eight eight-ounce glasses of water per day. (Be careful, however; too much water can result in water toxicity, so check with your doctor about your personal needs.) One way to test for adequate hydration is to check the color of your urine. It should be clear to pale yellow; a deeper yellow indicates that you are dehydrated and should be drinking more water.

*Caffeine.* Caffeine works as a diuretic, draining water from the body. It is also a stimulant, which may increase lid fissure width (vertical distance between upper and lower lids) in some patients, adding stress on the tear film by thinning and stretching the tear. It may also promote meibomian gland dysfunction. Cutting down on the number of cups of coffee, tea, or caffeinated cola drinks you consume each day, as well as the amount of chocolate you eat, can have a strong positive effect on dry eye symptoms.

*Vitamin Supplements.* Nutritional supplements especially designed to help dry eye are also on the market. These come under a number of brand names, including BioTears, TheraTears, and HydroEye, and are designed to stimulate tear production in order to reduce eye surface and gland inflammation. Most supplements come in capsules to be taken orally.

## About Over-the-Counter Eyedrops

Over-the-counter eyedrops are also known as artificial tears, but although they can provide relief, they cannot substitute for natural tears. Tears are complicated entities, and duplicating the complex arrangement of the three layers (lipid, water, and mucin) of natural tears is not really possible. Nevertheless, commercial eyedrops are more than simple saline solutions.

Artificial tears contain a viscosity-enhancing (mucin-replacement) component that allows them to adhere to the eye more effectively. The most common ingredient of this component is a cellulose compound, a type of polysaccharide. The cellulose compound swells up in water in order to retain moisture and adhere to the mucous membrane of the eye. Different brands of artificial tears use different types of cellulose at varying percentages to achieve varying levels of viscosity, depending on need. The higher the percentage of cellulose, the greater the viscosity and the longer the retention time of the artificial tears on the eye. (Higher viscosity drops tend to leave a "thready" residue on the lashes, which can be irritating although it is easily washed off with soap and water.)

Among the polysaccharides commonly used in artificial tears are hydroxypropyl methylcellulose (HPMC) and carboxymethylcellulose (CMC). Artificial tears also contain other minerals and elements found in natural tears.

Choosing among the myriad brands, types, and styles of over-the-counter eyedrops can be a bewildering process, and excellent new ones come on the market every year. Among those that I prescribe for aqueous tear deficient dry eye are the drops from the Refresh line (manufactured by Allergan). These range from Refresh Lubricant Eyedrops without cellulose (0% CMC, preservative free) to Refresh Tears (0.5% CMC), Refresh Plus Tears (0.5% CMC, preservative free), Refresh Liquigel (1% CMC), and Refresh Celluvisc (1% CMC, preservative free). Although they have the same percentage of cellulose, Celluvisc uses a higher-viscosity CMC and therefore is thicker—more viscous—than Liquigel and has a greater retention time.

Another line of tears I often recommend is Genteal (0.3% HPMC), Genteal Mild (0.2% HPMC), and Genteal gel. (These are manufactured by Novartis.) I also like the TheraTears line (manufactured by Advanced Vision Research), which are hypotonic. (TheraTears is 0.25% CMC and is also available as a gel.)

Hypotonic artificial tears have low salt concentrations, which help reduce the high salt concentrations that occur in dry eye states and that lead to surface inflammation. Hypotonic artificial tears have been shown to promote healing and reverse some effects of dry eye.

A relatively new drop liked by many patients is called Systane (Alcon). It was developed to strengthen the tear film by forming a soft gel matrix that adheres to the cornea, as opposed to simply replacing the tears. As a result, the artificial tears stay on the eye longer.

Another interesting new product is Nature's Tears EyeMist (Bio-LogicAqua Technologies), a nonallergenic eye spray that "penetrates" the tear film and thus increases the volume of tear film on the eye. Because it is a spray rather than a drop, it is easier for some patients to administer and can be used in most situations.

If meibomian gland dysfunction with lipid tear deficiency is diagnosed and evaporative dry eye is evident, I may recommend lipid or oil containing drops, such as Refresh Endura (which contains castor oil and glycerin) or Soothe Emollient Eye Drops (which contain mineral oil). These drops help stabilize the tear film.

### *About Preserved and Nonpreserved Eyedrops*

Preservatives are added to over-the-counter and prescription eyedrops to prevent contamination and to increase shelf life. Benzalkonium chloride (BAC) has the longest track record but is known to be irritating, causing toxic and allergic reactions in some users needing frequent eyedrops.

Many dry eye patients find they are especially sensitive to preservatives; some suffer more pain from using the preservative-containing artificial tears than from the dry eye itself. Fortunately, many artificial tears are now available without preservatives: examples are the single-use vial packs (Genteal PF, Refresh Plus Tears, Refresh Celluvisc) and the new multidose bottles (Visine Pure Tears) that make preservative-free drops more accessible and convenient. Other artificial tears contain gentle preservatives that dissolve when placed on the surface of the eye, thus reducing or eliminating the toxic effect. This includes sodium perborate found in Genteal and purite found in Refresh Tears and Liquigel.

### *Reducing Redness*

One of the most popular features of some over-the-counter eyedrops is their ability to reduce or eliminate redness in the eyes due to irritation from minor airborne pollutants (smoke, dust) or from allergens (pollen, ragweed, animal dander, grass). Among the more popular brands are Vasocon A, Naphcon A, and Visine (which currently offers several different products for redness relief, each with slightly different active ingredients to treat various symptoms).

The active ingredient that eliminates redness is called a vasoconstrictor. As with preservatives, different vasoconstrictors are used in different drops; among the more common are naphazoline, tetrahydrozoline, and oxymetazoline. Some drops that contain vasoconstrictors also contain a mild antihistamine (pheniramine maleate). Together these chemicals relieve many allergy symptoms: the antihistamines counteract the histamines that are released as the result of an allergic response, while the vasoconstrictors help relieve the redness and swelling in the eye's blood vessels and tissues caused by the body's reaction to the histamine.

Products containing vasoconstrictors can be problematic, especially for dry eye sufferers. Paradoxically, if overused, a vasoconstrictor can end up causing even more redness (a rebound effect), inflammation, and irritation as well as other even more serious problems such as increased blood pressure. Furthermore, reducing the redness may end up masking a more serious eye injury or disease.

I recommend that dry eye sufferers choose from among the

BOX 26

**Recommended Over-the-Counter Eyedrops, Gels, and Ointments**

Below is a list of products currently on the market that I recommend to my patients, and that they have found to be beneficial. The higher the percentage of cellulose (HPMC or CMC), the more viscous the drop. You may need to try various types to see which one works best for you.

Genteal Mild 0.2% HPMC; preservative
Genteal 0.3% HPMC; preservative
Genteal PF 0.3% HPMC; preservative-free single-use vials
Refresh Tears 0.5% CMC; preservative
Refresh Plus Tears 0.5% CMC; preservative-free single-use vials
Refresh Liquigel 1% CMC; preservative
Refresh Celluvisc 1% CMC; preservative-free single-use vials
Thera Tears 0.25% CMC, hypotonic; preservative; also preservative-free single-use vials
Systane Lubricant Eyedrops; preservative and preservative free
Systane Free Lubricant Eyedrops (gel); preservative
Refresh Endura (oil); preservative-free single-use vials
Soothe Emollient Eye Drops (oil); preservative
Refresh PM ointment 57.3% white petrolatum; mineral oil, preservative free
Tears Naturale PM ointment 94% white petrolatum; 3% mineral oil, preservative free
Genteal (gel); preservative

BOX 27

**The Art of Inserting Eyedrops**

Putting drops in your eyes effectively is actually not difficult, but a few pointers may help. The best way to insert drops—and keep them in your eyes—is to tilt your head back as far as you can, with your chin pointing toward the ceiling. Look way above your head. If you are right-handed, with your left index and middle fingers, pull down the lower lid of your eye, creating a little "pocket." (If you are left-handed, use your right index and middle fingers to pull down the lid.) With your opposite hand, gently squeeze the drops into the pocket, being sure not to touch your skin or your eyelashes with the dropper. Gently release the lid back into its normal position and blink two or three times to spread the drops over your eyes. Blot any excess liquid with a clean tissue. Repeat with the opposite eye.

drops I've suggested in Box 26. While soothing the underlying dry eye, these products may also help reduce or eliminate redness and inflammation.

### If Blepharitis or Meibomian Gland Dysfunction Is Present

Often with mild dry eye, posterior blepharitis or meibomian gland dysfunction may also be present—or even be the cause of the problem. These diseases cause inflammation of the eyelids and add to the dry eye pain. In addition to artificial tears, drops, or eye gels, you may want to try rinsing solutions, lid scrubs, warm compresses, or simple blink exercises (see Chapter 11).

For significant meibomian gland dysfunction, I often prescribe doxycyline, an antibiotic similar to tetracycline that is lipid soluble and gets into the meibomian glands to help reduce inflammation. Doxycycline not only kills bacteria, it also controls lipid inflammation within the glands.

Anterior blepharitis or infection of the lash follicles may also be present, adding to inflammation and other dry eye symptoms. The offender may be bacteria, a virus, a fungus, or even a parasite such as a mite called demodex. If the microbes are bacteria, treating your eyelashes with warm compresses and gentle scrubs made with diluted baby shampoo (one part shampoo to ten parts water) may help. Try not to get the shampoo in your eyes, as it could disrupt the tear film. After three to five strokes at the base of the eyelashes, rinse the lashes free of shampoo. If you don't experience improvement, your doctor may want to prescribe an antibiotic ophthalmic ointment.

## TREATING LEVEL 2 DRY EYE

Patients with moderate dry eye will have more symptoms than those with mild dry eye. Examination and testing will probably indicate a range of problems, including tear film instability with rapid breakup time and signs of inflammation. Also, patients may be experiencing blurred or fluctuating vision.

Unstable tear film can be the result of advanced aqueous tear deficiency (Schirmer testing will help determine its presence), or meibomian gland deficiency with lipid tear deficiency, or both. If patients have aqueous tear deficiency alone or coupled with meibomian gland deficiency, then therapies to increase the tear volume are recommended, including nonpreserved artificial tears, gels, topical steroids, cyclosporin A (Restasis), and secretagogues.

### Nonpreserved Artificial Tears and Gels

If little or no inflammation is present, patients may be treated with artificial tears; but because symptoms are more severe and more drops are needed throughout the day at Level 2, the drops should be nonpreserved to prevent preservative toxicity. For added relief, patients may also benefit from gels (such as Refresh Liquigel or Genteal gel), although these may transiently blur vision.

If using extra drops during the day is insufficient to relieve symptoms or signs of dryness, I would consider a punctal occlusion to preserve the few natural tears that are being secreted. Especially helpful when no significant inflammation is present, the occlusion can quickly provide comfort for moderate to severe symptoms in Level 2 dry eye.

If symptoms of dryness occur during the night or first thing in the morning, a nighttime ointment may be helpful, such as (preservative-free) Refresh PM ointment or Tears Naturale PM ointment, both of which contain white petroleum and mineral oil.

You may be sleeping with your eyes partially open, which allows the tears to dry up, a condition called nocturnal lagophthalmos. If so, the benefit of the bedtime ointment may be enhanced by using a plastic wrap (like saran) to create a humidified moisture chamber over your eyes while you are sleeping. Put ointment on the bony frame surrounding the eye, then place a piece of clean plastic wrap over the eye on the bony frame. The wrap will adhere to the ointment creating a humidified moisture chamber. Wear a sleep mask over the eyes to prevent dislodging the saran wrap.

Alternatively, irritation in the morning could be caused by blepharitis, floppy lid (where the upper lid inverts against the pillow), or recurrent erosion (where the lid sticks to the cornea and pulls off some epithelium). If floppy lid is the problem, wearing a patch over the lid while you sleep may provide relief. If you think the lid is sticking to the eyeball, gently massage the lid when you wake up to release it from the eye before opening your eye.

## Topical Steroids

If inflammation is present, depending on how severe it is, it may be treated with topical steroid drops, cyclosporin A (available as

BOX 28

**Case Study: Tom**

Tom was a 58-year-old newspaper journalist who worked hard (using his eyes extensively, often in front of a computer screen) and enjoyed lots of outdoor sports, such as golf, swimming, tennis, and skiing (all of which took their toll on his eyes). A doctor was treating him for ocular herpes of the right eye (herpes simplex of the cornea.) The eye was red, particularly painful, and nonresponsive to a topical antiviral medication for herpes simplex or to various antibiotic drops. The inflammation was not getting better; in fact, it seemed to be getting worse.

His doctor suggested that he consult with me on the off chance that he might have dry eye. I gave Tom a series of tests for dry eye, as well as for ocular herpes, just to be on the safe side. I determined that his herpes virus infection had subsided, but he did have a moderate to severe case of dry eye (Level 2, verging on Level 3). The tear clearance test showed moderate aqueous deficiency with delayed tear clearance. Also, it turned out that Tom suffered from mild rosacea and meibomian gland dysfunction.

I treated him with Lotemax, a topical steroid eyedrop, which he used for two weeks, together with an antiviral pill to prevent herpes simplex recurrences. I put him on a regimen of nonpreserved artificial tears, together with eye washes. Within a week, Tom's eye inflammation and his eye pain were gone. I took him off the Lotemax after the initial two weeks, but suggested that he continue using artificial tears as needed. Essentially, the various drops were irritating his dry eye, and the therapy required focusing on his tear deficiency.

Restasis), and/or oral tetracyclines (also doxycycline). It needs to be eliminated if at all possible, as it exacerbates dry eye symptoms and signs.

Steroids are a group of naturally occurring or synthetic organic compounds that include cholesterol, sex hormones, anabolic steroids, adrenocortical hormones, certain natural drugs, and the precursors of certain vitamins. Corticosteroids are the classic anti-inflammatory agents and eliminate virtually all aspects of inflammation.

Lotemax is the commercial name for a corticosteroid that is site specific; that is, it exerts its influence on the inflamed area, and then deactivates, thereby minimizing any adverse side effects, especially glaucoma and cataract. Lotemax reduces symptoms and signs of dry eye in patients with decreased tear clearance; I have also found it to be useful in patients with dry eye and inflammation even with normal tear clearance. Lotemax does contain a preservative, so your doctor will have to monitor you for any allergic or toxic response. Also, long-term use may ultimately cause cataracts and glaucoma and can predispose patients to infection.

## Cyclosporin A

Again, if inflammation is present—and it frequently is with moderate dry eye—patients can sometimes find relief with a prescription therapy known as cyclosporin ophthalmic emulsion 0.05%, known commercially as Restasis. This is the first prescription medication specifically developed for dry eye syndrome and it is quite popular.

Restasis is thought to help increase tears for people whose tear production is reduced because of inflammation on the surface of the eye and within the tear glands. It also diminishes inflammation in patients with moderate to severe dry eye and can help with dry-eye–related fluctuating vision. Restasis is not recommended if you have an eye infection or while you are wearing contact lenses. (If you use daily-wear contact lenses,

BOX 29

**Case Study: Carol**

Carol, a 52-year-old interior designer, came to see me with classic dry eye symptoms, especially a gravelly sensation in her eyes. Tests (Schirmer, TBUT), revealed aqueous tear deficient dry eye, plus erosions on her conjunctiva and cornea in both eyes.

Her symptoms were moderate compared to her signs. I placed her at Level 3, Severe Dry Eye, and recommended a punctal occlusion. However, she had heard about Restasis and was eager to try it, even though she understood that it might not reach full effect for about six months.

I put her on Restasis and nonpreserved artificial tears. The regimen didn't completely eradicate her symptoms, but it brought them under control and Carol was comfortable with the results. After several months her eyes showed reduced signs of dryness (to Level 2). I continue to monitor her to make sure her condition does not regress.

you can place the first drop in the morning fifteen minutes before inserting the lens and the second drop in the evening after removing the lens.)

Restasis can take up to six months to achieve full effect, so I often initially also prescribe Lotemax, which has a rapid onset of action, to quickly reduce any inflammation. Or a nonpreserved artificial tear can be used in conjunction with the Restasis until the Restasis itself takes effect.

## Secretagogues

Secretagogues are oral agents that cause or stimulate bodily secretions; they are most commonly used for patients with Sjögren's syndrome to increase saliva and tear production. Evoxac and Salagen are the best-known secretagogues and can be prescribed to help stimulate the lacrimal glands in dry eye patients. Their downside is that they may stimulate more tearing than is required, plus they may overstimulate the salivary or sweat glands. Other side effects may include headaches, intestinal cramping, and exacerbation of asthma.

### Punctal Plugs and Cautery

Sometimes artificial tears, ointments, and gels, as well as other topical medications, do not completely eliminate the pain experienced by a patient with dry eye. When these lubricating products simply do not bring sufficient relief, a punctal occlusion can be an effective alternative treatment.

Many doctors wait to perform a punctal occlusion until a patient's pain is quite severe (Level 3 or Level 4), but a punctal occlusion can provide relief very quickly and prevent symptoms from getting out of hand. One reason for holding back on this procedure is to avoid flooding a patient's eyes with toxic irritants and inflammatory mediators. However, I have found that if the inflammation is eliminated before the puncta are closed and if the eyes are rinsed regularly with sterile eye rinse, these irritants do not become a problem.

A punctal occlusion can be performed with punctal plugs or punctal cautery. Many punctal plugs are available; one type is a tiny silicone stopper that is inserted into the duct opening at the inner corner of each eye, thereby plugging the "drains" that normally allow tears to flow out of the eye and into the nose. Thus, even if tear flow is below normal, whatever tears are present remain longer in the eye.

Temporary (self-dissolving) plugs can be inserted to test if the occlusion will help; if they are successful, permanent (non-self-dissolving) plugs can then be inserted. Plugs can go into the upper or lower punctum, or both. However, plugs can sometimes be problematic: they can become dislodged and lost in the

BOX 30

**Case Study: Paula**

Paula, a banker in her late forties, came to me with a very obvious case of aqueous tear deficient dry eye. She was already at Level 3, Severe Dry Eye. She had had LASIK surgery, and as a result, one eye was very dry and her vision had suffered. She had already had her lower puncta occluded and had tried almost all the over-the-counter brands of artificial tears as well as Restasis, but her eyes were still irritated.

I decided that an upper punctal occlusion would be the quickest way to give Paula some relief. I cauterized (lightly) the upper puncta in her dry eye. Within a day or two, she was producing what turned out to be a slight excess of tears, although her eye was finally comfortable. The tears were welling up in her eye and at times would spill over onto her cheek. However, when I reopened her upper puncta slightly, within twenty-four hours she was absolutely normal. Her pain and excess tearing were virtually gone.

eye, cause a foreign body sensation and localized inflammation, or create an incomplete closure of the tear drain.

For this reason, I prefer punctal thermocautery, a minor procedure performed in minutes in the doctor's office. After numbing the lid around the puncta, the doctor cauterizes (seals off) the tear duct with a battery-operated, high-temperature wire. In many cases, I create a thin scar which can be easily reopened should the patient, for some reason, produce too many tears. (This scenario is more likely to occur if both the upper and lower ducts are closed.) Many patients have benefited from this approach. Other techniques have been developed to close the tear drains—including the use of radiofrequency needles, lasers, and sutures—but for me this one works best.

## TREATING LEVEL 3 DRY EYE

Dry eye patients at Level 3 experience painful and probably multiple symptoms most, if not all, of the time. Signs of corneal disease with early breakdown of the central cornea surface are present. Filamentary keratitis, a frustrating and painful disorder in which threadlike structures of mucus and degenerated cells attach to the cornea is a common problem. Every time you blink, you feel the filaments as they scrape the surface of the eye, creating a painful foreign body sensation.

Level 3 patients, like those at Level 2, may find relief with nonpreserved artificial tears, gels, ointments, as well as cyclosporin A (Restasis), topical steroids, oral secretagogue drugs, and punctal occlusion. In addition, the doctor may try a few other medications, including oral tetracyclines and/or autologous serum.

### Oral Tetracyclines

Tetracyclines (including doxycycline) are a group of antibiotic drugs commonly used to treat conditions such as acne, bronchitis, sexually transmitted diseases (syphilis, gonorrhea), as well as more obscure diseases such as Rocky Mountain spotted fever. With dry eye, tetracyclines are used to control and reduce inflammation on the ocular surface. Their anti-inflammatory properties also reduce inflammation within the meibomian glands.

### Autologous Serum

A unique eyedrop made from a patient's own blood, autologous serum contains various growth elements and anti-inflammatory factors normally found in natural tears and therefore deficient in patients who are not producing enough of their own tears. Also, these natural factors are not found in commercial eyedrops.

Autologous serum typically contains no preservatives and is soothing and nonirritating. Precisely because it contains no preservatives, it has the potential for contamination by microorganisms. Moreover, it is costly to make.

I process the patient's serum under sterile conditions in a certified laboratory in my office. A professional phlebotomist draws the blood from the patient. I let it clot, centrifuge it, then draw off the serum inside a sterile hood. I dilute it with sterile nonpreserved saline or tissue culture media, separate the lots into individual vials, then freeze them at minus 20 degrees Centrigrade. I dispense the serum drops to the patient. A vial lasts about ten days and must be refrigerated.

## TREATMENT OF LEVEL 4 DRY EYE

Patients with extremely severe dry eye are experiencing a sight-threatening disorder. Major breakdown of the corneal epithelium may be present, as well as other corneal troubles, including possible corneal ulcers. This level of dry eye is unusual and is generally associated with, or a manifestation of, a serious systemic autoimmune disease such as Sjögren's syndrome, Stevens-Johnson syndrome, or cicatricial pemphigoid.

Treatment for Level 4 can include any of the treatments previously listed for less serious dry eye, depending on the type of dry eye (aqueous tear deficient, evaporative) and other issues relevant to the patient (allergies or age, for example). Also, because extremely severe dry eye is usually tied to serious systemic diseases such as cicatricial pemphigoid, it can call for a number of more extreme forms of treatment including surgery.

### Systemic Anti-inflammatory Therapy

For very severe dry eye, systemic anti-inflammatory therapy may be required. This means that certain medications, including strong chemotherapeutic or immunosuppressive agents, may be taken systemically, usually orally. Ocular cicatricial pemphigoid is one of the most common diseases requiring this type of systemic treatment.

### Topical Vitamin-A Therapy

Dry eye resulting from serious illnesses (Stevens-Johnson syndrome) or disorders (ocular cicatricial pemphigoid) can make the conjunctiva and/or lid become extremely dry and scaly. A topical vitamin-A ointment, applied directly to the eyeball or the eyelid, can be highly effective.

### Acetylcysteine

Acetylcysteine is a drug used to dissolve mucus in various parts of the body, such as the chest in severe bronchitis and other pulmonary disease. Administered as an eyedrop, it can also be used to treat severe filamentary keratitis.

### Moisture Chamber Glasses or Goggles

Patients with dry eyes are troubled with air currents, especially from overhead fans, air conditioners, vents or open windows in a car, or air currents encountered when playing sports (riding a bicycle, water skiing, snow skiing, or any other sport where wind comes into the face). Patients with extremely severe dry eyes, as well as those with dry eye as a result of LASIK surgery or contact lens–related dry eye, may be helped by wearing specially engineered moisture goggles to protect their eyes, even for everyday use.

Moisture goggles are engineered to minimize evaporation of tears from the eyes of people with dry eye. A cross between goggles and sunglasses, most basic moisture goggles have a rubberized orbital seal that is fixed to a sort of sunglass frame, then covered with fleece, which absorbs moisture and prevents sweat from dripping into the eyes.

To eliminate potential fogging, some brands treat the inner surface of the lenses with an antifog treatment together with a tiny vent that allows a minimal amount of air to flow through. The frames wrap around the face, allowing both peripheral vision and a tight fit. Some moisture goggles can be equipped with prescription lenses, including bifocals. Some are purely therapeutic and look almost like swimming goggles, which makes wearing them during a normal workday not altogether desirable for patients concerned with their appearance. However, certain manufacturers such as Panoptx and Seefit (*www.panoptx.com* and *www.seefit.net*) have developed attractive—even fashionable—goggles that look very much like sunglasses.

## Surgery

A number of surgeries can be performed to help relieve more advanced cases of dry eye. These include punctal occlusion (including punctal cautery), ocular surface reconstruction, and various lid and lash surgeries. Surgeries for treating dry eye, like other surgical procedures, are relatively serious choices, but they can provide enormous relief.

### IF SURGERY IS REQUIRED

If your doctor recommends surgery to treat your dry eye, don't be alarmed. Several procedures are available today that are relatively routine to perform, are reasonably painless, and bring enormous relief for dry eye. A few of the more common ones are described below.

Although the Delphi panel table lists the surgery option for the most extreme cases of dry eye (Level 4), sometimes surgery may be useful at an earlier, less severe stage, such as dry eye symptoms from lid laxity.

Before you agree to any surgery, be sure you understand the operation itself as well as all issues surrounding the procedure as they pertain to your health and well-being, as well as to your dry

BOX 31

## Questions about Surgery for Dry Eye

Before you undergo surgery for dry eye, be sure to ask your doctor a lot of questions. If you are not sure you will comprehend everything he says, bring along your spouse or other family member or friend to take notes and/or ask additional questions. Below are a few general questions for you to consider.

**1** *What kind of surgery am I having? (Be sure to ask your doctor to describe it in detail.)*

**2** *How will the surgery affect my dry eye?*

**3** *How, if at all, will the surgery affect my overall vision?*

**4** *Why is the surgery recommended? What could I expect if I did not have the surgery?*

**5** *Will you be performing the surgery, or will it be another doctor? If another doctor, why? When and where can I consult with the surgeon?*

**6** *Will my surgery be performed in the doctor's office, or will I go to a same-day, outpatient surgicenter?*

**7** *How long will it take for my eye to heal?*

**8** *Will I have any restrictions after surgery?*

**9** *Will I experience much pain? If so, how will be the pain be handled?*

**10** *Is the procedure permanent? If not, when will my eyes return to normal?*

**11** *Will I be able to wear my contact lenses again soon? Will I be able to wear them again at all?*

eye. Consider the suggested questions in Box 31 and use them to create your own questions about your particular surgery.

## Punctal Occlusion

After eliminating inflammation, I often use punctal occlusion successfully in patients with moderate dry eye (Level 2) and reduced tear production, as well as in those with more severe dry eye. As described earlier, I prefer punctal cautery to punctal plugs. Either way, punctal occlusion is a routine procedure that often brings excellent results with regard to easing the pain of dry eye.

## Ocular Surface Reconstruction

Patients with ocular surface disorders, including conjunctivochalasis (where the conjunctiva loses its elasticity and creates folds that can hang over the lid margin), cornea ulcerations, Stevens-Johnson syndrome, ocular cicatricial pemphigoid, and chemical and thermal burns, may all benefit from ocular surface reconstruction using amniotic membrane grafting. First described in the 1940s, the procedure was not often used; however, advances in processing and preserving the amniotic membrane tissue have repopularized its use. It has enjoyed great success and usually allows for complete reconstruction of the ocular surface.

Human amniotic membrane is taken from a placenta obtained during elective (as opposed to emergency) Caesarean section, which has been washed and treated with medicine to prevent bacteria and fungal growth and preserved frozen at minus 80 degrees Centigrade. When needed, it is thawed and grafted onto the ocular surface, providing a foundation that promotes healing of damaged corneal and conjunctival surfaces while reducing scarring and inflammation.

The surgery is usually performed in a hospital or surgicenter, on an outpatient basis. The actual procedure is done under a microscope while the patient is under local anesthetic. The

BOX 32

**Case Study: Eloise**

Eloise is an accountant in her forties with two grown daughters. She wore soft daily-wear contact lenses for many years. Gradually, over a period of two years, she developed extreme dry eye pain. She stopped wearing her contacts, but her eyes remained irritated and uncomfortable. Actually, she was suffering from symptomatic conjunctivochalasis. After topical therapy failed to relieve her symptoms, I performed surface reconstruction using amniotic membrane on her more problematic eye. Within weeks she felt complete relief from irritation in that eye and could not wait to have the surgery on the other eye (which I performed sometime later). Ultimately Eloise was able to resume wearing her contact lenses comfortably.

patient can leave an hour or two after surgery. Healing time varies according to the disease being treated and the extensiveness of the damage to the eye, but typically within a few weeks the surgical graft is completely healed.

Although ocular surface reconstruction using amniotic membrane may be used for extremely severe, vision-threatening cases of dry eye (Stevens-Johnson syndrome, for example), I have also used it for more benign disorders, including symptomatic conjunctivochalasis. Although this disorder does not cause blindness, it can feature significant pain and suffering. The surgery has proved to be highly successful.

### Tarsorrhaphy

A tarsorrhaphy typically involves adhering (sewing) the outer eyelids or, less commonly, the inner upper and lower eyelids to narrow the eye opening and thus reduce the exposed ocular surface. The surgery is useful for patients who require ocular surface protection for an extended period or permanently. For example, patients suffering from Bell's palsy, stroke, corneal ulcers, Sjögren's syndrome, or severe dry eye may benefit.

Tarsorrhaphy is performed with local anesthesia in an operating room, a clinic, or your doctor's office. Stitches are placed at the outside corners of the lid opening. Because the eye opening is now smaller, the tear film is concentrated over a smaller exposed area, besides which the evaporation of tears is slowed because of the reduced surface area. Nevertheless, a regimen of eyedrops may still be necessary.

### Botulinum Toxin (Type A)

Botox, as it is commonly called, can provide a nonsurgical alternative to tarsorrhaphy. The same drug that is used for cosmetic purposes can be used to induce paralysis of the upper eyelid. The result is ptosis (droopy eyelid), which reduces exposure of the ocular surface. The ptosis will last about three months. However, Botox can also affect the lacrimal glands, resulting in a significant decrease in aqueous tear production, thus aggravating dry eye instead of helping to heal it.

Botulinum toxin (Type A) is also used successfully to relieve the forceful eyelid spasms in essential and secondary blepharospasm. Care is needed with this procedure to avoid excess weakening of the lid muscles, which could result in an inability to close the eyes.

### Trichiasis

Trichiasis is a disease in which the eyelashes become misdirected, growing inward toward the surface of the eye instead of outward. As a result, the sharp lashes can irritate or abrade the ocular surface. Trichiasis can be caused by chronic inflammation of the conjunctiva or eyelid, apparently leading to a mild scarring of the hair shafts that in turn leads to misdirection of the lashes. Even a single misdirected lash can not only cause incredible discomfort for a patient, it can lead to corneal ulceration and perforation.

The aberrant lashes can be dealt with simply by epilation or pulling them out. (Often patients do this on their own, but it is safer to have a doctor do it, to avoid scratching the ocular surface.) However, the hair follicle remains intact and the lash can grow back.

Procedures for permanently removing lashes include radiosurgical ablation, cryoepilation (freezing of the eyelid to kill the follicles), direct excision of the eyelash follicles, electrolysis, and laser ablation. Cryoepilation is effective, but frequently causes inflammation and scarring. Currently, radiosurgical ablation is the preferred technique: radiowaves are used to cauterize (and kill) each faulty eyelash follicle, and then the lash is removed.

## Other Possible Surgeries

Special surgery may be required for various problems of eyelid position such as lax, floppy, or droopy lids—in other words, problems that leave the surface of the eye vulnerable. Other possibilities are entropion (a rolling inward of the eyelid margin), ectropion (a rolling outward of the eyelid margin), and eyelid retraction (a pulling of the eyelid, exposing the surface of the eye).

CHAPTER

# 11

# Remedies for Home and Work

Myth

*Keeping dry eye syndrome under control is complicated and stressful.*

Fact

*Many small, simple changes can be made in your environment and lifestyle that will help enormously to keep the pain and irritation of dry eye in check.*

Dry eye often requires therapeutic measures that are almost as serious as the syndrome itself. Yet dry eye can also be controlled in a number of ways that are surprisingly simple and straightforward—maybe even fun. Easy-to-manage changes in your environment and your lifestyle can all lessen the pain and irritation of dry eye syndrome. Try a few of these; if necessary, try them all!

## YOUR ENVIRONMENT

The first element of your lifestyle that must be considered is the climate. Do you live in a moderate climate with changing seasons? If so, you need to think about how best to use fans and air conditioners during the hot months, and how to avoid blasts of heat and ultradry air when indoors—and minimize exposure to frigid, windy weather when outdoors during the cold months.

Do you live in a hot, sunny climate? If so, you may need to make sure you wear sunglasses whenever you are outside, and avoid the swirling air caused by fans or air conditioners, which can seriously affect your eyes.

Controlling your environment, whether it is in your house, in your place of work, in your automobile, or in any public place you frequently visit (your place of worship, a school, a mall, a restaurant), involves checking three basic elements: temperature, humidity, and lighting.

## Temperature

The temperature of most indoor or enclosed spaces is controlled by air conditioners, fans, or heaters—all of which pose problems for people with dry eye. In order to function properly, air conditioners and fans blow air in and around a room or space. This agitated air, which recirculates dust, pet dander, and other allergens and pollutants, not only irritates dry eyes but can make them even drier.

Air conditioning should be minimized. That being said (and I do live in Florida), I recognize that air conditioning is often imperative, especially on the hottest days. If you suffer from dry eye, make sure you are not sitting, standing, or sleeping in a place where an air-conditioning vent is blowing air directly at you, specifically at your face. Ceiling air-conditioning vents should be aimed up toward or parallel with the ceiling, not downward toward the floor. Also, louvers of window air-conditioning units should not be directed toward the middle of the room, but upward toward the ceiling. The same holds for air circulated by a ceiling fan, as it will cause the tear film to evaporate too quickly, even sometimes while you are asleep. So minimize ceiling fan use, or better yet, avoid it.

Heaters, in some cases, also blow dry air around a room. That air is warm or hot, exacerbating dry eye even more. Heat originating from fireplaces and wood-burning stoves is equally problematic for dry eye sufferers, especially since it is coupled with smoke. Again, avoid direct contact with hot air or smoke as much as you possibly can.

## Humidity

Humidity is another environmental factor that needs to be considered and controlled. If you live in a very dry climate or if the indoor air in your home or workplace is particularly dry, especially during colder months, invest in humidifiers, especially for the bedroom, office, and any other space where you spend a considerable amount of time (see Box 33).

## Lighting

Lighting is another critical element to be considered by dry eye sufferers, both in the home and at the office. Our eyes need adequate light to work, but as a dry eye sufferer you may paradoxically need more light (especially if you are over age 65) at certain times and less light at others.

Bright light, including sunlight, can irritate dry eyes (a problem called photophobia) and cause sufferers to squint or close their eyes for comfort. Fluorescent lights can also aggravate dry eyes. To minimize symptoms, use artificial tears regularly. At the same time, reduce the wattage of the light bulbs in your home or office, use direct task lighting, and try special lenses in your glasses that will automatically increase their tint in brighter light.

## Stop Smoking!

I know you have heard it a million times—but I'm going to say it again: Smoking—of cigarettes (including low tar), cigars, or pipes—is very damaging to your health. It causes lung cancer, emphysema, heart disease, and bronchitis, and contributes to many, many other maladies, one of which is dry eye syndrome.

Studies have shown that cigarette smoke is not only irritat-

BOX 33

## About Humidifiers

Humidifiers are almost a requirement for anyone suffering from dry eye. They can ease the pain and help keep the eyes moist. They also help hydrate dry skin and relieve other problems resulting from dry air. Anyone who suffers from dry eye (as well as dry throat or dry skin) can benefit. Humidifiers relieve sinus pressure and sinus headaches, help alleviate sinus infections, and keep nasal passages from drying out.

Many brands and styles are available, including tabletop (which suffice for a single room), console (which come with larger tanks, enough to humidify several rooms), and whole-house humidifiers (which are actually considered the most efficient and quiet, and are the least expensive to operate.) Tiny, portable ultrasonic humidifiers can be useful in small nooks around the house, in the car, or on airplanes or in hotel rooms, especially in rooms where you cannot otherwise control the heat and humidity.

The most significant element in any humidifier is the humidistat, which controls the humidity level and shuts off the device when the desired level is reached. (Indoor humidity should be 40 to 55 percent; overhumidifying a space can cause condensation and lead to growth of mold or bacteria.)

Humidifers also come in "warm mist" styles (with a tiny heater that warms the water before it is put into the air) or "cool mist" (equipped to blow cool, misty air into the environment.) Some humidifiers are both air purifiers and humidifiers, and allow the user to turn off the humidifier when it is not needed but keep the purifier on full time. A humidifier-purifier can be a boon for dry eye sufferers or anyone with severe allergies.

ing, but also alters or disturbs all three layers of normal tear film: the mucin secretion from the conjunctival goblet cells, the watery secretion from the lacrimal glands, and the lipids from the meibomian glands. Moreover, it decreases tear breakup time. Even nonsmokers are susceptible when exposed to secondhand smoke.

If you smoke and suffer from dry eye, here is my prescription: Quit smoking immediately. If others in your household smoke, urge them to quit smoking as well, and in the meantime ask them to smoke outdoors. There is no risk-free level of exposure to secondhand smoke, according to the new Surgeon General's scientific report released June 27, 2006. Not only does secondhand smoke aggravate your dry eye, it is virtually as deadly as firsthand smoke.

## Controlling Your Home Environment

Taking precautions to protect your eyes inside your home is both easy and incredibly helpful. Check the temperature, humidity, and lighting in all the rooms of your house, and pay special attention to the bedroom, the kitchen, the home study, and the workshop and/or garage. When you clean, follow the tips in Box 34.

### *The Bedroom*

The bedroom is probably the most important room in the house for keeping dry eye controls in place. It is the room where you spend the greatest amount of time, and since much of that time is when you are asleep, it is imperative that you have all your "dry eye controls" in place.

These days it is fashionable—even economical—to install overhead fans in summer houses and homes in warmer climates. Still, no matter how fashionable or cost efficient a ceiling fan may be, avoid using one, most particularly in the bedroom. In addition to causing pain, the agitated air can dry out tear film (even when the eyes are thought to be closed in sleep), thereby initiating dry eye syndrome or aggravating existing dry eye. If you must, substitute small table or floor fans, and place them so that they are blowing away from you.

Minimize the use of air conditioning in the bedroom, if possible. If you must use it during the hottest days, as with a fan, be sure the air vent is directed upward toward the ceiling or horizontally along the ceiling.

Bedding (bedspreads, comforters, and the like) can harbor mites, microbes, and other allergens that exacerbate allergies and possibly cause dry eye. To keep bedrooms as allergy free as possible, use throw rugs instead of wall-to-wall carpeting; wash bedding and rugs frequently in hot water and dry them in a hot dryer. (Check the manufacturer's label for special cleaning instructions.)

### *Kitchen and Dining Areas*

The biggest culprits in the kitchen and dining areas are related to smoke. Dry eye sufferers need to avoid smoke, which can be incredibly painful and may profoundly exacerbate existing dry eye. If you are the primary cook, avoid frying or other smoky cooking techniques, use an exhaust fan, and leave the kitchen if someone else is cooking.

As delightful as candlelight is, lighted candles should be avoided on your dining table.

### *Home Study*

Your home office should be as efficient and "dry eye friendly" as your place of work, especially with regard to lighting and your computer. This is important whether you go online once a month to pay bills or spend many hours every day working (or playing) on the computer or reading. For details about setting up a computer in an ideal office, see the section on computer vision syndrome.

BOX 34

**House-Cleaning Tips**

Many cleaning products and techniques wreak havoc on dry eye sufferers, especially if the dry eye is associated with allergies. Here are a few practical suggestions:

- Never combine ammonia and bleach. Together, the chemicals are highly combustible and can literally burn your eyes.
- Avoid aerosol cleaning sprays. Instead, use a plain nonspray product, or take off the nozzle and apply the product with a cloth or paper towel.
- Be very careful with powdered cleaners; use liquid cleaners (nonspray!) instead.
- For dusting, use a damp cloth or paper towel to remove dust. Wipe down surfaces that won't be damaged with a very mild alcohol-water or bleach-water solution, which will also help keep mold and mildew under control.
- Use microfiltration bags or electrostatic filters in your vacuum cleaner. These filters cost more than the standard ones and may fit only certain vacuum cleaner models, but they work better at trapping small particles. For the most effective removal of allergens, buy a vacuum cleaner with a HEPA (high-efficiency particulate arresting) filter, a type of filter found in the best air purifiers.
- Keep dust cloths and other cleaning cloths clean. Wash them frequently in hot water and bleach to make sure you are not recycling microbes, mites, or other allergens. Never use a feather duster; it simply flicks dust into the air and thus into your eyes.

- If your eyes are extremely sensitive to dust and other airborne materials, wear goggles when you clean house.
- Consider wearing a surgeon-type mask over your nose and mouth when you are cleaning. Such masks can be purchased at most drugstores.
- Change the filter in your air conditioner at least once a month during times of heavy use.
- Use air purifiers (with HEPA filters) in rooms where you spend the most time, especially the bedroom.
- Wear gloves while you clean, and keep your hands away from your face.

### *Workshop and Garage*

Avoid engines that burn diesel fuel in machines large and small. Use a hand-powered lawn mower, and don't use a leaf blower or other machine that blows dry, hot, or toxic air into your eyes. Wear goggles, especially when you are working with drills, saws, or any other tool that might endanger your eyes.

## Your Car

Your car is another environment that needs to be controlled if you suffer from dry eye. Also, you should exercise certain precautions with regard to driving to protect yourself from exacerbating existing dry eye, or possibly developing dry eye.

### *Circulating Air*

One of the biggest problems in your car is circulating air. If it is hot outside, the problem is the air conditioner or open windows; if it is cold, the problem may be the car's heater. In either case, as always, try to keep circulating air to a minimum

BOX 35

**Controlling Dry Eye in Your House: A Checklist**

This checklist will help you ensure that your house is as dry eye friendly as possible.

- In the bedroom, avoid using ceiling fans, particularly directly over the bed.
- If you use floor or table fans or air conditioning in your bedroom, make sure the air is directed away from the bed, specifically away from your face and eyes.
- Use a humidifier in the bedroom, particularly if you live in a dry climate and during the winter months when the indoor air tends to be excessively dry.
- Put small humidifiers in other rooms where you spend a considerable amount of time, or invest in a whole-house humidifer.
- To avoid mites or microbes that might cause allergies, wash throw rugs, comforters, and blankets frequently in very hot water and dry them in a hot dryer. (Always check the manufacturer's cleaning label.)
- In the bathroom, don't use heaters, especially those that circulate air around the room.
- Don't burn candles in the bathroom or bedroom, on a dining table, or anywhere where smoke can affect dry eyes.
- Avoid hair dryers, and never point one directly at your eyes.
- Evaluate your home computer setup, and make sure it is optimal.

- Check the lighting in every room in the house to be sure it is direct and appropriate in places where you are using your eyes: in the kitchen when you are cooking, in your home office or study, and near chairs where you read or do other close work such as knitting, embroidery, painting, or woodwork.

and avoid aiming the air conditioner or the heater directly at your face.

If your car's air conditioner seems to be making you sneeze, the culprit may be fungi that produce airborne mold spores and can grow within the air-conditioning system. To minimize this problem, keep the car windows open partway for about ten minutes after you turn on the air conditioning and never direct the vents toward your face. If these steps don't help, have your car's air-conditioning system cleaned and treated with a disinfectant that is available at car dealers, service stations, and car repair shops.

Circulating air is, of course, a supreme problem in convertibles. As a dry eye sufferer, avoid riding in convertibles; if you must do so, wear sunglasses or even moisture chamber goggles.

### *Driving Tips*

The other problem with automobiles and dry eye is long-term driving. The effect of driving for hours on end is much the same as long-term reading, long-term knitting, long-term computer work—or any other activity in which you stare at something for long periods. The prolonged staring profoundly affects your blink rate, and the tear film dries up.

When driving, practice the following:

Wear sunglasses, especially in bright light.
Rehydrate frequently. Stop for water, or keep bottled water handy.
Stop every half hour and stretch your body, especially your neck, back, and shoulders.
Massage your scalp to relax muscles in your head and neck.
Exercise your eye muscles by looking far left, right, up, down; focus on something close up, then on something far away.
Use lubricating eyedrops every hour.
Blink frequently—at least every ten seconds.

## Controlling Your Work Environment

At home, you have the freedom to arrange your environment to suit your wants and needs. That is not always true in an office, factory, studio, or other place of work. In fact, usually you have very little control over environmental factors at work. Other "powers-that-be" stipulate how close to or how far from a window you work, whether a heat or air-conditioning duct is located directly over your desk, and whether your office is inordinately hot or cold, dry or humid. In addition, perhaps your workplace, for whatever reason, is subject to fumes that might cause an allergic response that could lead to irritation and dry eye symptoms. You can still take a number of steps to make your workplace safe and healthy, especially if you suffer from dry eye (see Box 36).

### *Talk to Your Boss*

I believe that it is critical for dry eye sufferers to inform their bosses about their disease. For starters, given the symptoms of dry eye (redness in the eyes, inflammation, constant blinking, inappropriate tearing), your superior may think you are spending your nights out on the town, drinking excessively or taking

BOX 36

**Improving Your Workplace: A Checklist**

Make a close inspection of your office or everyday workstation, the place where you spend most of your workday. After you have checked for possible factors that may aggravate your dry eye, discuss them with your superior and work together to remedy as many of the problems as possible.

Air-conditioning vents. Check the location of any vents near your desk. If one is blowing excessive air in your face throughout the day, ask to have it closed, covered over, or redirected.

Overhead fans. Make sure your desk or workstation is not located directly under a ceiling fan. If it is, ask to have that particular fan turned off.

Heating ducts. Be sure heating ducts are not located in such a way that the heat is blowing directly into your face and eyes. If so, ask that it be closed. Ask if you can use a small space heater instead.

Lighting. Check out the lighting in your office or workstation. If the overhead lighting is too harsh and glaring, turn it off (if you control it) or ask if it can be turned off—or if a few of the bulbs or fluorescent tubes can be removed. If the natural light is too harsh, ask to have the blinds pulled. At the same time, make sure that localized lighting for detailed work (such as computer or other close work) is strong enough.

Fumes. If you work in a factory, a restaurant, a hospital, or any other venue where fumes can be a problem, determine that exhaust fans and other air purifiers are in place. Wear moisture goggles if necessary, and irrigate your eyes with eye rinses.

Smoke. Many businesses now demand that their offices be smoke free. If smoking is permitted in your place of work, ask that your office or workstation be in a designated smoke-free zone, or at least apart from smokers.

Special eyewear. If you have severe dry eye, you may want to consider wearing moisture chamber goggles. (This decision, of course, depends on the severity of your dry eye and the conditions of your workplace.)

drugs, and wonder if your partying is affecting your work. Even if she understands that you have a problem with your eyes, she might wonder if you can be productive if you are in such pain.

I recommend that you make an appointment to talk with your boss in detail about dry eye in general, your dry eye problems, and what you are doing to resolve them. Together the two of you can then optimize your work environment so that you (and your eyes) are as comfortable as possible.

For example, you might be able to close an air-conditioning vent that blows irritating air in your face, or redirect a heater that spews unwelcome hot air into your office. Harsh lighting can be problematic. Your boss may be able to turn off certain fixtures—or at least remove a few bulbs—that directly impact your comfort level and order eye-easing task lamps for your work area. If you currently sit near someone who smokes, perhaps your desk, workstation, or office can be moved.

### *If You Work in a Factory*

Depending on the industry, many factories have firm individual safety guidelines. If you suffer from dry eye, avoid dirty, dusty, or moldy conditions as much as possible. If you cannot stay away from these conditions completely, wear moisture chamber goggles at all times, irrigate your eyes regularly, and of course follow to the letter all safety measures required by the law and by your particular business.

## COMPUTER VISION SYNDROME

Over the past twenty years, computers have become as much a part of our lives as television sets and telephones—perhaps even more so. At work and at home, many of us spend hours in front of a computer screen either doing our work (more than 75 percent of office jobs require a computer these days) or paying bills, emailing friends and family, and playing computer games.

More and more people are experiencing eye problems related to excessive computer use. These include eyestrain, undue fatigue, burning sensation, irritation, redness, and blurred or double vision.

The scientific community has labeled this complex of symptoms "computer vision syndrome" and has discovered that by far the most prevalent contributor to the problem is dry eye. Indeed, many of the factors characterizing computer vision syndrome are identical to the elements that define classic dry eye syndrome. These include:

*Environmental factors.* Many offices generate factors that play havoc with vision and induce eye irritation: dry air, problematic heating and air-conditioning systems, building contaminants, plus dust and other allergens and toxins related to paper, toner, and office tools and supplies.

*Reduced blink rate.* Studies have shown that blink rates among computer users are severely reduced, which leads to increased tear evaporation and poor tear film quality, with stress on the cornea and symptoms of dry eye.

*Increased ocular exposure.* With normal reading, the upper eyelid covers much of the eyeball, minimizing evaporation of tear film. During computer work the user is normally viewing the material horizontally, not downward; the result is a wider lid fissure that increases exposure and evaporation.

*Contact lens use.* Many office workers wear contact lenses, and it has been determined that those who also spend long hours in front of a computer screen are likely to suffer a higher level of eye strain and irritation than non–contact lens wearers. Also, if the surface of the eye is dry, the lens sticks to the eye during a normal blink, resulting in intense discomfort.

## Treating Computer Vision Syndrome

As with dry eye syndrome in general, treating computer vision syndrome requires a multifaceted approach. The computer user's work environment is involved, and certain eye therapy measures need to be taken.

*Lighting.* Improper lighting conditions within a workstation can affect a computer user's eye comfort. Surrounding sources of light, especially overhead fluorescent lighting, large windows, and poorly placed desk lamps can create glare, which in turn can cause eyestrain. If possible, to correct these problems turn off harsh lights or remove a few of the bulbs; place blinds or tints on the windows; if necessary, move the workstation to another location. For task lighting, choose ordinary incandescent bulbs that are "warmer" and cause less glare, making them easier on the eyes. Aim for a consistent level of brightness, and avoid bright and dim spots or shadows.

*The computer screen or monitor.* Computer vision syndrome seems to be directly related to the quality and design of the screen or monitor; the more frequently the screen refreshes itself, the clearer the image. Look for refresh rates of at least 300 hertz to help provide a clearer image. Liquid crystal displays (LCDs) generally have high refresh rates and are well tolerated. A high-density dot matrix (90 dots per inch or greater) with dark characters against a light background produces a sharper image on the screen, which, not surprisingly, is easier on the eyes. Fortunately, the quality of monitors is getting better and better; if you are working with a monitor that is more than four years old, you might consider buying a new one. Also, an antiglare filter will reduce and improve contrast on the screen.

*Positioning of the screen.* Some studies have shown that the screen should be 16 to 30 inches from the user, while other studies indicate that distances from 35 to 40 inches may ease visual strain. Find the distance that is most comfortable for you.

More important, the screen should be placed 10 to 20 degrees (that is, the middle of the screen should be 5 or 6 inches) below eye level. Higher screens not only create eyestrain (because more of the eyeball is exposed, leading to rapid tear evaporation) but also cause strain on the back and neck muscles.

*Computer eyeglasses.* If you work in front of a computer more than three hours a day, it may be worthwhile to invest in glasses that you use solely for computer work. Occupational progressive lenses are available, providing a broad space at the top of the lenses for computer screen work (middistance viewing) and a second lens for close-up work, such as reading or keyboarding.

*Lubricating drops.* If you suffer from dry eye, you are probably using drops already. Even if you are not in the throes of dry eye, but you still work several hours each day in front of a computer, using over-the-counter eyedrops every couple of hours can help lubricate the ocular surface and maintain an optimum tear film. Some studies indicate that higher-viscosity eyedrops are more beneficial; however, they may affect your visual acuity.

*Mini breaks.* It used to be standard practice for workers to have a fifteen-minute break in the morning, another in the afternoon, and an hour for lunch. Before the advent of the computer, office workers actually would have several natural breaks, in that they would, for example, type a letter, get up to file, move back to the desk, and turn to answer the telephone. Working at a computer (which often includes email communications instead of the "old-fashioned" telephone messages) demands long periods without significant movement. Frequent short breaks (a walk around the office, a short stroll to get a drink of water, just leaning back and closing your eyes) are imperative. You might want to try a few blink exercises as well or apply a compress to your eyes.

## YOUR DIET

Not surprisingly, excellent ocular health is directly related to the quality of your diet. Maintaining your proper weight, getting sufficient sleep, eating a balanced and healthy diet, all have a profound impact on the health of your eyes and the treatment of your dry eye. Indeed, the Delphi panel judges dietary issues to be among the first facets to be considered when treating dry eye.

In addition to a healthy, well-balanced diet, a few dietary factors are crucial for keeping dry eye in check. Although these were discussed in Chapter 10, it is worth mentioning them again.

*Increase your water intake.* Experts have found that simply by increasing the amount of water consumed every day, dry eye symptoms may be controlled. A healthy diet includes about eight eight-ounce glasses of water per day.

*Reduce caffeine.* Caffeine works as a diuretic and drains water from the body. Cutting down on the number of cups of coffee, tea, or caffeinated cola drinks you consume each day, as well as amount of chocolate you eat, can have a strong effect on dry eye symptoms. Caffeine is also a stimulant and may increase lid fissure width in some patients; it may also promote meibomian gland dysfunction.

It is best to avoid caffeine altogether, or limit it to one day per week. If you must have it daily, use caffeine-free (or if necessary, decaffeinated) products and/or limit yourself to one cup of coffee or tea (or cola) per day. To maintain hydration, you might consider drinking a glass of water after you've had a cup of coffee or tea.

*Eat more fish.* A recent study found that adding tuna fish (at least five servings per week) to the diet was effective in reducing

BOX 37

**Easy Ways to Add Fish to Your Diet**

Many people, especially those living in land-locked regions, find that buying and preparing fish dishes can be a problem. Many people find cooking fresh fish difficult, or they don't like the smell. Fortunately, two of the fish highest in omega-3 fatty acids are tuna and salmon, both of which are available in cans. Select the tuna canned in water. Tuna canned in oil may not have as many omega-3 fatty acids because the oil (soy or vegetable) can leach some of the natural tuna oil out of the tuna. Here are a few suggestions to help you get at least five servings of fish into your diet per week, even if you live in rural Kansas.

- Eat a tuna fish sandwich (on whole wheat bread, with a minimum of low-fat mayonnaise) for lunch once or twice a week.
- Add a small (three-ounce) can of tuna or salmon to a green salad for a nutritious lunch.
- Make a big batch of old-fashioned tuna-noodle casserole. (Go heavy on the tuna, light on the low-fat cream sauce.) It's great comfort food.
- Order a tuna, salmon, or mackerel entrée when you eat in a restaurant. Most restaurants—even steak houses—offer grilled tuna or salmon as alternatives to beef.
- Dine occasionally in a Japanese restaurant, choosing a tuna or salmon entrée (teriyaki, for example). Try sushi or sashimi at least once! It's delicious.
- To keep fishy smells out of the house, prepare tuna, salmon, or mackerel steaks on an outdoor grill. (As a dry eye sufferer, if you are the cook, be sure the grill is covered as the fish cooks.)

the rate of dry eye in women. Tuna is very rich in omega-3 fatty acids, which seem to stimulate healthy lipid and aqueous tear production. Other excellent choices are salmon, mackerel, and sardines. (The best fish nutritionally are wild as opposed to farm raised.)

*Take flaxseed oil every day.* Flaxseed oil has become a major factor in the treatment of dry eye, primarily because it is another incredibly rich source of omega-3 fatty acids. Flaxseed oil can be purchased in health food stores, in seed, capsule, or liquid form. It tends to oxidize rather quickly (especially the liquid) and must be kept refrigerated in an airtight container. If it tastes or smells bad, it has turned rancid and should be thrown out. A common dosage is one to two tablespoons of flaxseed oil or one or two flaxseed capsules per day. It can be consumed "straight" (like cough medicine) or mixed with fruit, yogurt, smoothies, or protein drinks.

*Take nutritional supplements.* Vitamins and other nutritional supplements can be helpful for dry eye sufferers, and supplements especially designed to ease dry eye are readily available. These come under a number of brand names, including BioTears, TheraTears, and HydroEye, and are designed to stimulate tear production in order to reduce eye surface and gland inflammation. Most supplements come as capsules that are taken orally.

## SPORTS

One of the principal factors in maintaining excellent health is keeping active. Certainly, one of the best ways to make sure that your body is exercising properly is to participate in sports. But for dry eye sufferers, taking part in many common sports can be excruciatingly painful, to the point where participation is either limited or must be stopped. Any sport that involves wind circulating around the face is problematic. And, of course, with wind come increased amounts of dust, sand, or splashing water. Many outdoor sports require coping with intense sunshine, which also can aggravate dry eye. Think about it: Such diverse sports as bicycling, in-line skating, ice skating, skiing, sailing, waterskiing, and even running, all involve wind blowing against the face and eyes and often require coping with other elements as well, including intense sunshine, glare, and water or rain.

Dry eye sufferers, even those with just a mild case, should get in the habit of wearing sunglasses (preferably large-frame wraparounds) at all times. If your dry eye is moderate to severe, invest in goggles and wear them religiously when participating in sports. Some sports, such as skiing, offer a line of goggles appropriate to the sport. However, moisture goggles, even if they are not fashionable, should be worn if your ski goggles do not keep your eyes moist. Dry eye sufferers should take the following additional precautions, depending on their sport:

If possible, wear a hat with a broad brim (a sun hat, a baseball cap) to provide further protection from the sun.
Wear a sweatband to prevent salty sweat from dripping into your eyes.
Lubricate your eyes with artificial tears every few hours.
Drink lots of water; stay hydrated.
Blink frequently.

## PROPER EYE CARE

The easiest way to avoid eye pain is to get in the habit of protecting your eyes as much as possible all the time. This is especially true when you suffer from dry eye as well as frequent eye infections, eye allergies, or other eye diseases and disorders.

### Basic Eye Hygiene

Avoid touching your eyes as much as possible. Some people who suffer from dry eye develop the habit of constantly rubbing their eyes. Not only does the rubbing tend to increase inflammation, it also can allow microbes to enter the eye, possibly leading to infection. Some people use a soiled handkerchief or tissue to rub their eyes; avoid this practice as well.

When you must touch your eyes (to put in drops or insert your contact lenses, for example), be sure your hands are clean. Wash your hands with a fragrance-free soap (Dove for sensitive skin) and then rinse them thoroughly. Some people find the humidity of a shower or bath comforting for their dry eye; but when washing your hair, don't let the shampoo flow over your eyes, and use a hypoallergenic, fragrance-free shampoo.

*Rinsing solutions.* Using sterile 0.9% saline solution or an over-the-counter eye rinse, flush your eyes each morning immediately after getting out of bed and at the end of the day. For relief during the day, especially if you have been reading, driving, or working at a computer, you may want to rinse your eyes again.

*Eye scrubs.* If you are suffering from meibomian gland disease or blepharitis in addition to dry eye, clean your eyes daily with an eye scrub. Scrubs are available commercially (Novartis Eye Scrub and OcuSoft Lid Scrubs are two recommended brands) and are premoistened cleansing pads.

To make your own simple scrub: In the palm of your clean hand, mix a small drop of baby shampoo with warm water in a ratio of about 1:10. With a cotton swab or your clean fingertip, brush the edges of the upper and lower eyelids at the base of the lashes with the shampoo solution several times, then rinse it off. Try to keep the shampoo out of your eyes. If you also have a prescribed ointment, use it after the lids are scrubbed.

### Makeup and Other Beauty Products

Choose hypoallergenic makeup, particularly any cosmetic that comes in contact with your eyes. This includes face creams and lotions, face powders, and, of course, eye makeup such as eye shadow, eye liner, and mascara. With a non–oil-based makeup remover, clean your face before going to bed. Apply makeup carefully and in moderation, as some will inevitably make its way into the tear film, potentially irritating the eye. If you are suffering from moderate to severe dry eye, forgo using eye makeup altogether until your dry eye is under control.

Use fragrance-free soaps, body lotions, and shampoos. Avoid hair spray and nail polish of any kind, if possible, until your dry eye symptoms are under control.

### Glasses and Sunglasses

Make sure the prescription for your glasses is up to date. If it is not current, your vision may be blurry and the blurriness may lead to increased staring, which can worsen dry eye symptoms. Unfortunately, until the dry eye is under control it is impossible to get a completely accurate prescription.

Get into the habit of wearing ultraviolet blocking sunglasses whenever you are outside. Invest in a suitable pair of wraparound sunglasses, to give you added protection from bright light. If you wear spectacles, get prescription sunglasses.

### Warm Compresses

Get into the habit of soothing your eyes with warm compresses. Not only is a warm compress soothing, but it loosens lash deposits so that the eyes are more easily kept clean. The heat from a compress also helps to "melt" abnormally thick meibomian gland secretion, allowing it to flow more readily onto the lid margin.

Eye compresses can be made in several ways. You can simply soak a clean washcloth in hot water (but not so hot that it will scald your skin), then apply it to your eye for several minutes. Patients of mine are using some interesting alternatives: they fill a clean sock with raw rice and microwave it until the rice is hot but not scalding (about a minute), or they put a clean baked potato in the microwave, warm it, then place it on the eye. Both techniques create "formed" compresses that fit comfortably in the socket of the eye.

### Blink Exercises

Exercising the eyes with conscious blinking is helpful in stimulating and spreading tears across the eyes adequately. If you have a partial or inadequate blink, try practicing in front of a mirror. Remember, with a good blink, the lids should touch before opening. Blink gently ten times, then repeat the exercise three times. Also, if you have been focusing on one object (a computer screen, a book, a road), consciously focus on something completely opposite. (For example, if you are doing close work, focus on something distant; if you are driving, focus on something close up.)

Perform these exercises several times during the day. Try to remember to do them before your eyes begin to feel fatigued or irritated.

### Eye Breaks

Perhaps the best thing you can do for your eyes is merely to close them. Several times during the day, take a deep breath, add an artificial tear, then close your eyes and leave them closed for a minute or two. This will revive your eyes, your energy level, and even your spirits.

CHAPTER

# 12

# Twenty Frequently Asked Questions

Myth

*Dry eye syndrome is a rare phenomenon, and we needn't worry about it.*

Fact

*Close to 10 percent of the industrialized world may suffer from dry eye syndrome, causing significant loss of productivity in the workplace and much personal suffering, pain, and even loss of vision.*

I am constantly asked questions about dry eye syndrome, not only by my patients but by friends, acquaintances, and even medical colleagues. I can think of no better way to end this book than to answer the twenty most common questions I am asked about dry eye. Here they are.

**1** *What is dry eye syndrome?*

Dry eye syndrome, or keratoconjunctivitis sicca, is a condition where the cornea and conjunctiva of the eye are excessively dry because of abnormal tears, leading to damage to the eye's surface. There are two types: aqueous tear deficient dry eye, caused by problems with the lacrimal glands; and evaporative dry eye, usually the result of problems with the meibomian glands. Symptoms include burning, itching, grittiness, and foreign body sensation in the eyes, with frequent redness and inflammation.

**2** *Are dry eye syndrome and dysfunctional tear syndrome the same thing?*
Yes, they are. In recent years, scientists have been leaning toward the latter, because the name more clearly reflects the complexity of the disorder.

**3** *Is dry eye syndrome a serious disease?*
Absolutely. Although in its early stages it may seem like a minor irritation that can be treated with over-the-counter eyedrops, it can escalate quickly. It will not clear up on its own, like a cold. In fact, left untreated it can result in blindness in severe cases.

**4** *I have heard that one's environment plays a major role in dry eye syndrome. Is this true? If so, how?*
Environment is one of the primary factors affecting the development, exacerbation, and healing of dry eye. However, environment refers not simply to the local climate—although that does play a part. Dry eye is affected also by the microenvironments of the home, workplace, automobile, and any other place where a dry eye sufferer spends a lot of time.

Further, an environment may not simply need to be "dry" to cause dry eye. In fact, the disease often has more to do with circulating air from air conditioners and heaters, as well as the presence of allergens and other toxins. Environment is one of the primary factors that require acknowledgment and control in order to heal dry eye.

**5** *Can wearing contact lenses cause dry eye?*
In some cases, yes. Prolonged contact lens wear cuts down on corneal sensitivity; tears are not stimulated properly and dry eye can result.

**6** *If I am diagnosed with dry eye syndrome, does that mean I can never wear contacts again?*
You *may* be able to wear contacts after developing dry eye. However, you must first resolve the dry eye problem and then select the proper contact lenses.

**7** *Can working long hours at a computer cause dry eye?*
Yes. People who spend long periods staring at a computer screen may end up not blinking with sufficient frequency to lubricate the eye surface. Over time, computer vision syndrome and/or dry eye syndrome may result. The same is true of people who watch television frequently, sew or read for long periods, or spend many hours driving. In other words, any long-term activity that demands intense staring and not blinking frequently may result in dry eye.

**8** *Does LASIK surgery cause dry eye syndrome?*
LASIK surgery may cause dry eye, and a significant number of people who have had the surgery develop at least transient dry eye. The most common explanation is that the corneal nerves are cut during LASIK surgery and thus no longer participate in the integrated circuit responsible for producing healthy tears.

**9** *I suffer from hay fever and often have itchy, irritated eyes during allergy season. Is my allergy related to dry eye syndrome?*
Possibly, as a dry eye cannot clear allergens from its surface and is unable to adequately dilute any allergens that get in the eye. Also, the medication (that is, the antihistamine) you use to treat your hay fever may lead to dry eye or exacerbate existing mild dry eye.

**10** *I have heard that dry eye syndrome is a geriatric disease—that only older people get it. Is that true?*
The answer is both no and yes. Dry eye can develop for reasons having nothing to do with advanced age (prolonged contact lens wear, allergies, and so on) and therefore can be found in people of all ages. Nevertheless, the greatest number of dry eye sufferers are women over the age of 50. This may have to do with the decreased production of the androgen hormone as a result of menopause. Also, certain geriatric diseases, including Parkinson's disease, are related to dry eye.

**11** *Is it true that dry eye syndrome is mainly a female problem, that only women get it?*
Yes, it is true that most people (over 60 percent) who suffer from dry eye are women. However, many men, particularly older men, suffer from it too.

**12** *Why do more women than men suffer from dry eye syndrome?*
The development of dry eye in menopausal women may have to do with the depletion of the androgen hormone. Paradoxically, androgen is primarily a male hormone; men have much more of it, and although they also lose androgen, they do so much more slowly. As a result, dry eye shows up predominantly in women, particularly menopausal women.

**13** *I have heard that dry eye syndrome is associated with some serious diseases. What are they?*
Dry eye syndrome is related to a number of very serious autoimmune diseases, including Sjögren's syndrome, diabetes, lupus, rheumatoid arthritis, and Graves' disease. Dry eye is also associated with Stevens-Johnson syndrome, rosacea, and Parkinson's.

**14** *If my eyes are dry and irritated, will commercial, over-the-counter eyedrops solve the problem?*
Yes and no. In some cases, over-the-counter drops will be sufficiently comforting. In other cases, using over-the-counter products can exacerbate the problem. Many commercial eyedrops contain preservatives, which cause an irritation or burning sensation and can be toxic (that is, damage the surface cells of the cornea) in some eyes.

**15** *I've tried using several different over-the-counter eyedrops to ease my irritated eyes, but none of them seem to work. Is there anything further I can do?*
Yes, there are several avenues you should explore. First, you may be allergic or sensitive to over-the-counter preservatives; try a preservative-free drop. Also, your pain and irritation may be a moderate to severe case of dry eye, demanding more than

simple eyedrop therapy. Consult a reputable eye doctor as soon as possible.

**16** *I've heard that Restasis is the cure-all for dry eye. Is that correct?*
Restasis is the brand name for cyclosporin A, and it has enjoyed a lot of publicity and a certain amount of popularity. The first drug developed specifically for dry eye syndrome, it is aimed at reducing the surface inflammation that exacerbates dry eye. Although it can be useful therapy, it is not a cure-all. Since Restasis is a prescription drug, you need to consult with your eye doctor in order to get it. He or she may well include additional therapies with the Restasis.

**17** *I have heard about special glasses or goggles for dry eye. What are these?*
Special moisture chamber goggles have long been recommended for dry eye sufferers. Today a number of attractive types are on the market. Also, if you use a computer more than three hours a day, I strongly recommend that you be fitted with glasses for use only when you are at the computer. Computer glasses can ease eye strain and help prevent dry eye.

**18** *Are there any home remedies that can ease the irritation and pain of dry eye syndrome?*
Yes, a number of home remedies can ease dry eye pain. Most involve controlling your environment, both at home and at work. Certain scrubs, soothing compresses, and natural remedies are available as well.

**19** *Do I need to see a doctor if I suspect that I have dry eye syndrome? If so, what kind of doctor?*
If you suspect you have dry eye syndrome, I strongly recommend that you see an experienced eye doctor. Dry eye syndrome can be a tricky problem. At times, the pain can be rather extreme, but the exam findings of dry eye disease may be minimal. Conversely, because the surface can become numbed owing to lack of tears, the exam findings of dry eye disease may be much

more serious than your symptoms indicate. It is important that an eye doctor take a close look: see your optometrist or a general ophthalmologist. If the condition is severe, you may need to see a specialist, usually an ophthalmologist who has received special training in ocular surface disease, dry eye, or corneal diseases and surgery.

**20** *Is dry eye syndrome a chronic disease? Or can I be cured?*
The answer depends on how you define "cured." If, for you, cured means that you no longer need to rely on tear supplements and can ignore all environmental conditions because they no longer affect your eye comfort, then I would have to say that dry eye is a chronic disease, unlikely to be cured. However, dry eye can be managed to achieve absolute comfort and stop further damage to the eyes; in that sense it *can* be cured.

# GLOSSARY

NOTE: All terms are defined here as they relate to dry eye.

ABSORPTION The process by which tear components are taken back into or used by the body.
ACETYLCYSTEINE A drug used to dissolve mucus in various parts of the body; may be used to treat severe filamentary keratitis.
ACINUS One of the tiny sacs in the meibomian glands that synthesize the meibomian gland lipids.
ALLERGEN A substance that when introduced into the body stimulates an allergic reaction.
ALLERGIC REACTION A complicated chemical response to the presence of an allergen in the body.
ALLERGY An acquired sensitivity to certain substances, such as plants, pollens, or drugs, that may include such symptoms as sneezing, runny nose, red or inflamed eyes, and rash.
AMBLYOPIA Commonly referred to as lazy eye.
ANDROGEN A steroid that controls the development and maintenance of masculine characteristics, such as facial and body hair, and the development of the penis. Androgens also support various glands, including the tear glands. In women, the ovaries secrete small amounts of androgens until menopause.
ANTERIOR BASEMENT MEMBRANE DYSTROPHY A condition in which an irregular corneal surface can lead to dry eye when the overlying tear film becomes unstable.
ANTERIOR BLEPHARITIS, see also **blepharitis**. An inflammation of the eyelash follicles, usually from a bacterial infection, with crusting and flaking around the lash root.
ANTERIOR CHAMBER The space between the cornea and the iris, filled with a fluid that nourishes eye cells.

ANTIBODY A protein substance produced in the tissues of the body in response to the presence of an antigen (a toxin, for example), destroying or weakening it and thus creating the basis for immunity.

ANTIDEPRESSANT A drug used to prevent or relieve depression.

ANTIGEN A substance such as a bacterium, toxin, or microbe, that when introduced into the body stimulates the production of antibodies.

ANTIHISTAMINE One of several drugs used to counteract the physiological effects of histamine.

AQUEOUS HUMOR The transparent fluid within the anterior chamber of the eye that nourishes the cells inside the eye, controlling eye cell growth and maturation.

AQUEOUS TEAR DEFICIENT DRY EYE A form of dry eye that occurs when the lacrimal glands fail to produce watery tears.

AQUEOUS TEAR LAYER The middle, watery layer of the tear film. Composed mostly of various proteins, electrolytes, sugars, and water, and secreted primarily by the lacrimal gland.

ARTIFICIAL TEAR A fluid prepared to supplement inadequate tear production in dry eye patients. May also be used to relieve mild discomfort caused by drying irritants such as wind, smoke, or dust.

ASTHMA A condition in which the airways (mouth, throat, windpipe, lungs) are swollen and narrowed because of hypersensitivity to certain stimuli, including pollen, smoke, or even cold air.

ASTIGMATISM A defect of vision, usually due to an irregularly shaped cornea.

ATOPIC KERATOCONJUNCTIVITIS A chronic, severe allergic reaction to pollen, animal dander, and other substances usually affecting middle-aged men. If advanced, can cause scarring of the cornea and even blindness.

AUTOLOGOUS SERUM A unique eyedrop made from a patient's own blood.

BANDAGE CONTACT LENS A contact lens used on damaged or postoperative eyes to promote healing and protect the corneal surface.

BELL'S PALSY Paralysis or weakness of the facial muscles due to a malfunction of cranial or facial nerves.

BLACK EYE A bruising around the eye together with broken blood vessels in the white of the eye and swelling of the lid and tissue around the eye.

BLEPHARITIS An inflammatory condition that affects the edges of the eyelids, possibly with scales, crusts, shallow ulcers, or inflamed oil glands, causing itching, burning, pain, and redness on the surface of the eye. **Anterior blepharitis** usually refers to a bacterial infection of the lash follicles; **posterior blepharitis** is caused by a malfunction of the meibomian glands and is also called **meibomian gland dysfunction.**

BLINK A usually involuntary movement of the eyelid that distributes the tear film over the surface of the eye.

BOSTON SCLERAL LENS The commercial name for a special contact lens that rests on the sclera, clear of the cornea, allowing a diseased or damaged cornea to stay moist and protected.

BOTULINUM TOXIN, TYPE A (also **Botox**) The same drug that is used for cosmetic purposes; a nonsurgical alternative to tarsorrhaphy inducing paralysis of the upper eyelid, resulting in ptosis that reduces exposure of the ocular surface.

CATARACT A clouding of the eye's lens, or the part of the eye responsible for focusing light on the retina.

CELLULOSE COMPOUND A type of polysaccharide that swells in water in order to retain moisture; used in artificial tears in varying amounts, resulting in different degrees of viscosity.

CHALAZION A small bump in the eyelid caused by obstruction of the oil-producing meibomian gland.

CHEMICAL BURN A damaging irritation caused by exposure to a chemical (acid or lye, for instance).

CHOROID (also **choroid coat**) A vascular tissue containing large, pigmented cells that lies between the retina and the sclera and helps provide nutrients to the outer retina.

CICATRICIAL PEMPHIGOID A chronic autoimmune disease that features scarring of the conjunctiva and at times other mucosal tissues in the nose, throat, esophagus, urethra, vagina, and anus. The scarring can lead to obstruction of the lacrimal or meibomian glands and destruction of the goblet cells of the conjunctiva, resulting in tear instability and dry eye.

CILIARY BODY The intraocular tissue behind the lens responsible for secreting aqueous humor.

COMPLETE ANDROGEN INSENSITIVITY SYNDROME (CAIs) The syndrome in which a mutation in the androgen receptor gene leaves the body unable to respond to the androgen hormone, often leading to dry eye.

COMPUTERIZED TOMOGRAPHY A computerized imaging test using radiation that can check for lacrimal gland enlargement, growths, or tumors behind the eye.

CONJUNCTIVA The transparent membrane that lines the inner eyelid and covers the front of the eyeball (the sclera) except over the cornea.

CONJUNCTIVITIS (also **pink eye**) An inflammation of the conjunctiva, the outermost layer of the eye that covers the sclera, characterized by redness and sometimes accompanied by a discharge.

CONJUNCTIVOCHALASIS A common disorder in which the conjunctiva loses its elasticity, becomes wrinkled or pleated, droops over the lid margin, and becomes pinched between the lid and the eyeball, causing pain. Left unchecked, it can lead to dry eye and even tearing.

CONTACT CONJUNCTIVITIS A common allergic response to an allergen that has been introduced directly onto the eye such as an eyedrop, or a cosmetic such as eyeliner.

CONTACT LENS A plastic or polymer disk that is placed directly onto the eye to correct refractive vision disorders (nearsightedness, farsightedness, astigmatism).

CONTRAST SENSITIVITY A feature of vision whereby everything looks crisp, colorful, and clear. When reduced, everything looks washed out or overexposed.

CORNEA The transparent dime-sized front of the eye, sometimes called the window of the eye; with the lens, allows the eye to focus.

CORNEAL EPITHELIUM The most superficial cells covering the corneal surface, several cell layers thick.
CROCODILE TEAR The kind of hypocritical or fake tear often produced by a recalcitrant child. Also, the liquid (probably closely related to saliva) flowing from the eye of a real crocodile as it stalks and eats its prey.
CYCLOSPORIN, see also **Restasis**. An immunosuppressant drug produced by a fungus, sometimes used to inhibit organ transplant rejection.

DACROCYSTITIS An infection of the tear sac that lies between the inner corner of the eyelids and the nose.
DECONGESTANT A medication, often found in over-the-counter as well as prescription drugs, that breaks up congestion in the sinuses or chest by reducing swelling.
DELAYED TEAR CLEARANCE Improper drainage of tears, sometimes caused by a clogged tear duct, which can cause inflammation of the eye surface.
DELPHI CONSENSUS APPROACH A scientific method of collecting information from a field of experts on a particular subject. Seeks to define treatment of dry eye syndrome based on its severity.
DERMATITIS (also **eczema**) Inflammation of the upper layers of the skin causing itching, redness, swelling, and scaling.
DETACHED RETINA, see **retinal detachment**
DIABETES A serious but common disorder in which the pancreas produces insufficient or no insulin. Often involves eye problems, which can include dry eye syndrome.
DISTRIBUTION The manner in which tears are spread across the cornea and drained from the eye through the tear drainage system into the nose.
DIURETIC A substance or drug that tends to augment urination; causes the body to eliminate water. May cause dry eye through decreased watery tear production.
DROOPY EYELID, see **ptosis**
DRY EYE SYNDROME Known formally as **keratoconjunctivitis**

**sicca.** Characterized by faulty production of tears resulting in damage to the surface of the eye and at times painful eyes.

ECTROPION The condition in which the eyelid turns away from the eyeball and fails to cover the eye properly, leaving the eye exposed and potentially dry.
ECZEMA, see **dermatitis**
EDEMA The accumulation of excessive water in cells or tissues or body cavities.
ENDOTHELIUM The single layer of cells lining the inner cornea that keeps the cornea from swelling by removing excess water.
ENTROPION The condition in which the eyelid turns inward; often associated with eyelashes rubbing against the eye (trichiasis).
EPI-LASIK A surgical procedure closely related to LASIK and used to correct refractive vision problems. Only surface epithelium, not deeper corneal tissue, is cut before applying the laser.
EPISCLERA The connective tissue between the conjunctiva and the sclera.
EPISCLERITIS Inflammation of the episclera.
EPITHELIUM Tissue that makes up the covering of most of the surfaces of the body, including the eyes.
ESSENTIAL BLEPHAROSPASM An involuntary neurologic disorder usually in patients over 60 years of age, where the eyelids and sometimes the facial muscles spasm. The spasm may cause irritation.
ESTROGEN Any of several substances (hormones) secreted by the ovary and placenta that stimulate the female secondary sex characteristics.
ETIOLOGY The cause of a disease or abnormal condition.
EVAPORATION The rate at which tears are converted into vapor after they are secreted and distributed onto the surface of the eye.
EVAPORATIVE DRY EYE A form of dry eye syndrome characterized by an abnormal tear composition because of insufficient oil production by the meibomian glands; results in overly rapid evaporation of tear film.
EXCIMER LASER A special laser used to perform LASIK surgery.

EYE (also **eyeball**) The organ of sight. A spherical, hollow organ lined with a vast variety of cells, including those of the cornea, lens, and retina.
EYEBROW The bony ridge over the eyes as well as the hair growing on there. Together with the eyelashes, protects the eye.
EYELASH The fringe of hair at the edge of the eyelid. Designed to catch airborne particles before they enter the eyes.
EYELID The moveable fold of skin, muscle, and glandular tissue that can be closed over the eyeball.
EYE MUSCLE One of several small muscles on the outside of the eye, which allow the eye to move.

FARSIGHTEDNESS (also **hyperopia**) The condition that occurs when the light entering the eye focuses behind the retina, instead of directly on it. Objects seen at close range are blurry.
FILAMENTARY KERATITIS A disorder where stringy filaments of mucus are found attached to the cornea, creating pain, redness, and fluctuating vision.
FLAXSEED OIL A vegetable oil high in omega-3 fatty acids; seems to help reduce dry eye.
FLOATER Cellular material that floats in the vitreous humor in front of the retina. Usually harmless, but can indicate a tear or detachment of the retina.
FLOPPY EYELID SYNDROME A disorder characterized by lax or flaccid upper eyelids.
FLUORESCEIN An orange-red compound that exhibits intense yet harmless fluorescence (an emission of electromagnetic radiation); used in ophthalmology to reveal corneal lesions.
FOREIGN BODY SENSATION The feeling that an object—a fleck of dust, an eyelash, a wood sliver—has lodged in the eye, causing irritation or pain.
FOVEA The depression in the center of the retina made up only of cone cells; the most sensitive part of the eye.

GIANT PAPILLARY CONJUNCTIVITIS (GPC) A disorder affecting people who wear contact lenses. Features "giant papillae," or bumps of swollen tissue, with a central dilated vessel on the lining of the upper eyelid, making contact lens wear difficult or impossible.

GLAND A cell or group of cells, or an organ, that selectively removes material from the blood, concentrates or alters it as necessary, and secretes it for further use by the body or eliminates it from the body.

GLAUCOMA A blinding disease caused by elevated intraocular pressure that usually results from inadequate functioning of the eye's internal fluid drainage structures.

GEL A suspension of fine particles that have combined in such a way as to produce a semisolid, often oily material. Used to treat dry eye.

GOBLET EPITHELIAL CELL A conjunctival cell that produces mucin for the tear film, which in turn enables the watery tear film to adhere to the eye surface.

GRAFT-VERSUS-HOST DISEASE A post–bone-marrow-transplant incompatibility reaction against the host; this reaction may cause dry eye.

GRAVES' DISEASE A condition caused by excessive thyroid hormone; sometimes characterized by an enlarged thyroid gland, protrusion of the eyeballs, rapid heartbeat, and nervousness.

HERPES KERATITIS (also **ocular herpes**) A type of corneal infection brought on by the herpes simplex virus. Symptoms may include blurred vision, sensitivity to light, redness, pain, and disruption of the blink reflex.

HERPES SIMPLEX A common virus that affects the skin, mucous membranes, nervous system, and eyes.

HIV-AIDS Acquired immunodeficiency syndrome that is associated with dry eye syndrome from aqueous tear deficiency.

HORMONE REPLACEMENT THERAPY (HRT) The administration of estrogen and other hormones to menopausal women, usually in order to reduce osteoporosis and hot flashes.

HYPEROPIA, see **farsightedness**

HYPHEMA Bleeding in the anterior chamber of the eye.

HYPOTONIC ARTIFICIAL TEAR Having lower than normal salt concentration and, as a result, healing and soothing to dry eye sufferers who tend to have tears with high-salt concentrations.

IMBRICATION OF LIDS An overlapping of the upper and lower lids where they meet at the outer corner of the eye. This overlapping may cause irritation that may be confused with dry eye.

IRIS The colored part of the eye, which expands and contracts in order to control the amount of light coming through the pupil and into the eye.

KERATITIS Inflammation of the cornea.

KERATOCONUS A degenerative disease of the cornea that causes it to gradually thin and bulge into a cone-like shape.

LACRIMAL APPARATUS The tear production and drainage system consisting of tear glands, lid puncta, tear drainage ducts, collection sac within the nose, and duct from the sac to the internal lining of the nose.

LACRIMAL CANALICULUS One of the tear drainage ducts leading from the lid puncta to the collection sac inside the nose.

LACRIMAL FUNCTIONAL UNIT The integrated tear secretory system whereby tear gland secretion and eyelid blink are stimulated by the sensory nerves on the surface of the cornea through a reflex within the spinal cord.

LACRIMAL GLAND A gland under the conjunctiva in the upper outer corner of the eye that produces watery tears.

LAGOPHTHALMOS A condition in which the eyelids do not close completely; **noctural lagophthalmos** occurs when the eyelids do not close completely during sleep.

LASEK (laser subepithelial keratomileusis) A variation of PRK; a surgical technique to treat refractive disorders.

LASIK (laser in situ keratomileusis) A common refractive procedure used to correct nearsightedness, farsightedness, and astigmatism; the nerve endings are cut or ablated to reconfigure the cornea.

LAZY EYE, see **amblyopia**

LENS (also **crystalline lens**) The internal optical component of the

eye, responsible for adjusting focus; elastic and transparent. Located behind the iris and suspended on fibers from the ciliary body.
LID FISSURE WIDTH The vertical distance between the upper and lower lid margins. May cause dry eye syndrome when increased.
LID LAXITY A condition in which the lower lid does not properly hug or cover the eyeball. Usually age related, and closely associated with ectropion.
LIPID LAYER The oily, outer layer of the tear film, made up of waxy meibum produced by the meibomian glands.
LISSAMINE GREEN TEST A standard dye test given to dry eye patients to determine whether the epithelial cells are degenerating.
LUPUS ERYTHEMATOSUS An autoimmune disorder in which the body's immune system attacks tissues and organ systems throughout the body, causing inflammation. The skin is often involved; a red, blotchy, butterfly-shaped rash on the cheeks and bridge of the nose is common.
LYSOZYME An antibacterial agent found in tears, which in a matter of minutes inactivates bacteria on the surface of the eye.

MACULA The center of the retina; responsible for central vision (as opposed to peripheral vision).
MACULAR DEGENERATION (also **age-related macular degeneration**) A degenerative condition of the macula.
MACULAR EDEMA (also **cystoid macular edema**) A swelling of the macula, typically as a result of disease, injury, or eye surgery.
MAST CELL A type of cell found in connective tissue (mucous membranes, lung tissue, conjunctiva, nose) that contains numerous basophilic granules and releases substances such as heparin and histamine in response to injury or inflammation of bodily tissue. Often associated with allergies.
MAST CELL STABILIZER A type of drug that inhibits mast cells, preventing them from releasing allergic substances.
MEIBOMIAN GLAND A sebaceous gland in the eyelid that produces oil for the lipid layer of normal tear film.

MEIBOMIAN GLAND DYSFUNCTION A condition in which abnormally functioning meibomian glands result in lid inflammation and an abnormal lipid tear layer. Common cause of dry eye syndrome.
MEIBUM A complex mix of lipids, consisting of wax and sterol esters, hydrocarbons, triglycerides, free sterols, free fatty acids, and polar lipids; secreted by the meibomian glands.
MICROKERATOME A special cutting instrument for lifting the epithelial and stromal flap during LASIK surgery.
MOISTURE CHAMBER GLASSES OR GOGGLES Special eye protectors engineered to minimize evaporation of tears in dry eye sufferers.
MRI (magnetic resonance imaging) An imaging test using strong magnetic fields that can check for lacrimal gland enlargement or growths and tumors behind the eye, as well as for Graves' disease.
MUCIN A glycoprotein, mucus-like substance produced by the goblet cells of the epithelial layer of the conjunctiva.
MUCIN LAYER The layer of the tear film that lies closest to the surface of the eye; stabilizes the tear film and helps to spread tears across the cornea.
MYOPIA, see **nearsightedness**

NEARSIGHTEDNESS (also **myopia**) A common eye problem that occurs when light entering the eye focuses in front of the retina instead of directly on it. Objects far away are blurry.
NONPRESERVED EYEDROPS (also **nonpreserved artificial tear**) A drop or artificial tear that does not contain any chemicals to keep it contamination free.
NON-SJÖGREN'S AQUEOUS TEAR DEFICIENCY, see **primary acquired lacrimal gland disease**

OCULAR ALLERGY An allergy involving the eye.
OCULAR HERPES, see **herpes keratitis**
OCULAR ROSACEA An eye problem typically characterized by meibomian gland dysfunction, and surface and corneal inflammation associated with a chronic skin condition known as rosacea.

OCULAR SURFACE DISEASE INDEX © A respected medical test designed to assess the degree to which a patient has developed dry eye syndrome.

OINTMENT A semisolid, highly viscous preparation often containing medicine; usually meant to be applied externally.

OMEGA-3 FATTY ACID Any of various polyunsaturated fatty acids found primarily in fish, fish oils, vegetables, and vegetable oils (including flaxseed oil); thought to reduce dry eye.

OPHTHALMOLOGIST A physician who specializes in care of the eyes. Conducts examinations to determine the quality of vision and the need for corrective glasses. Checks for presence of eye diseases or disorders such as glaucoma and cataracts, as well as associated systemic medical diseases. May prescribe glasses, medication, or perform surgery, as necessary.

OPHTHALMOLOGY The study of the eye; the diagnosis and medical and surgical treatment of all diseases and disorders that affect the eye.

OPTICIAN A person who fills prescriptions for ophthalmic lenses and dispenses eyeglasses.

OPTOMETRIST A specialist trained to examine the eyes, check for the presence of eye diseases, and prescribe, supply, and adjust glasses or contact lenses. A graduate of optometry school, not medical school. Cannot prescribe all drugs and cannot perform surgery.

OPTOMETRY The practice of assessing vision, diagnosing eye diseases and disorders, and nonsurgically treating general eye problems as well as establishing whether glasses or contact lenses are needed to correct a visual defect.

ORBIT, see **socket**

PARKINSON'S DISEASE A usually geriatric disease that involves the nervous system and the destruction of brain cells, and features chronic tremors, slow movement, possible facial paralysis, and general weakness. Does not cause dry eye, but often associated with it.

PATHOGENESIS The development of a disease or morbid condition.

PATHOGENIC Having the capability of causing disease; producing disease.

PERENNIAL CONJUNCTIVITIS An ocular allergy that is present year-round and involves sensitivity to dust, plants, indoor molds, and other perennial allergens.

PERIMENOPAUSE The transition period of reduced ovarian function, associated with irregular menstruation and dry eye, that precedes menopause.

PHOTOABLATION LASER PROCEDURE Laser surgery on the cornea of the eye, as in LASIK and other refractive eye surgeries.

PHOTOPHOBIA A sensitivity to bright lights.

PINGUECULA A benign, yellowish degenerative growth that can form on the conjunctiva of the eye.

PINK EYE, see **conjunctivitis**

POSTERIOR BLEPHARITIS (also **meibomian gland dysfunction**), see also **blepharitis**. Inflammation of the meibomian glands, causing them to stop producing sufficient meibum or tear lipids.

POSTERIOR CHAMBER The area behind the iris where the lens of the eye is located.

PRESBYOPIA A condition of the eye in which the natural lens has become rigid and can no longer focus easily on near objects. Common among adults over age 40.

PRESERVATIVE A substance such as benzalkonium chloride that is added to artificial tears and other eyedrops, inhibiting contamination and giving them a longer shelf life. Can exacerbate pain and irritation in dry eye sufferers.

PRIMARY ACQUIRED LACRIMAL GLAND DISEASE (also **non-Sjögren's aqueous tear deficiency**) The most common cause of dry eye syndrome, involving a breakdown of the functioning of the lacrimal glands, which fail to produce sufficient aqueous tears.

PRK (also **photorefractive keratectomy**) A refractive surgical procedure whereby a laser is used to ablate the surface epithelium of the cornea. Unlike LASIK, no flap is cut on the surface of the cornea.

PSEUDOPEMPHIGOID Abnormal scarring of the ocular surface conjunctiva from chronic use of certain topical glaucoma medications.
PTERYGIUM A raised, wedge-shaped growth of the conjunctiva onto the cornea.
PTOSIS (also **droopy eyelid**) A sagging of the eyelid that may occur as a result of disease, injury, birth defect, eye surgery, or age.
PUNCTAL OCCLUSION A surgical procedure whereby the puncta are surgically closed either with plugs or by cautery.
PUNCTUM A small hole at the inner corner of the eye that permits tears to drain into the nose. Each eye has an upper and a lower punctum.
PUPIL The black "dot" at the center of the iris; actually a hole through which light travels to the retina.

RECTUS MUSCLE One of six muscles that attach to the outside of the eye, to move the eye.
RECURRENT EROSION SYNDROME A periodic breakdown of the corneal epithelium in which the lids pull a thin layer of cells off the cornea; typically causes acute sharp pain on opening the eyes when awakening.
REFRACTIVE SURGERY One of the surgical procedures—LASIK, LASEK, PRK, and epi-LASIK—used to correct refractive eye problems, such as nearsightedness, farsightedness, and astigmatism.
RESTASIS Commercial brand name for cyclosporin A (cyclosporin ophthalmic emulsion 0.05%), an eyedrop especially created to treat dry eye. Can reduce inflammation, thereby allowing the lacrimal glands to produce additional aqueous tears.
RETINA The ten-layer "film" at the back of the eye that records light; includes rod cells (that respond to light) and cone cells (that respond to color).
RETINAL DETACHMENT (also **detached retina**) A serious eye disorder that involves detachment of the sensory layer of the retina from the pigment layer; can lead to permanent blindness.
RHEUMATOID ARTHRITIS An autoimmune disorder that affects joints of the fingers, wrists, toes, and other body joints, making

them swollen, stiff, painful, and sometimes deformed. Often seen in conjunction with Sjögren's syndrome; thus, the lacrimal and saliva glands may also be affected.

RHINITIS Inflammation of the nasal mucous membranes; symptoms include runny nose.

RIGID GAS-PERMEABLE CONTACT LENS A type of contact lens that is rigid or firm.

ROD CELL A cell in the retina that responds to light.

ROSACEA (also **acne rosacea**) A chronic skin condition of the face, especially the nose and cheeks, characterized by dark rose skin coloration together with deep-seated pustules, resulting in an acne-like appearance. Can be associated with ocular rosacea, which in turn can evolve into severe dry eye.

ROSE BENGAL TEST An evaluation using rose bengal, a red dye, to assess the health of the conjunctiva epithelial cells, specifically which cells are inadequately coated with mucin.

SARCOIDOSIS A disease of unknown origin marked by formation of inflammatory lesions in tissues throughout the body, including the lacrimal gland, and causing dry eye.

SCHIRMER TEST A method of assessing tear production and helping to determine and treat dry eye syndrome.

SCLERA The dense white outer coat of the eye, enclosing the eyeball except for the part covered by the cornea.

SCLERITIS An inflammatory disease that affects the conjunctiva, sclera, and episclera.

SEASONAL CONJUNCTIVITIS The most frequent form of ocular allergy; a response to allergens released into the air at certain times of the year (as pollen in the spring).

SEBORRHEIC LID DISEASE A type of meibomian gland dysfunction with excess lipid secretion.

SECONDARY BLEPHAROSPASM Frequent blinking or actual spasm of the eyelids, caused by dry eye irritation. The eyelid spasm may further increase irritation, causing a cycle of more forceful spasms. Compare with **essential blepharospasm.**

SECONDARY LACRIMAL GLAND DISEASES Various disorders, including sarcoidosis, graft-versus-host disease, and HIV-AIDS, that can affect the functioning of the lacrimal glands.

SECRETAGOGUE A hormone or other agent that stimulates secretion; used orally for moderate to severe cases of dry eye syndrome.

SJÖGREN'S SYNDROME A condition in which the secretory glands, most commonly the lacrimal gland of the eyes and salivary glands of the mouth, are gradually destroyed by autoimmune inflammation leading to excessively dry eyes and mouth. May occur in conjunction with other autoimmune disorders, such as rheumatoid arthritis or systemic lupus erythematosus.

SLITLAMP A type of biomicroscope used to view the condition of the surface of the eye.

SOCKET (also **orbit**) The bony structure formed by the brow, the cheekbone, and the bridge of the nose that holds and protects the eyeball.

SOFT CONTACT LENS The general name for a type of contact lens made of a soft, malleable polymer. Styles include daily wear (removed nightly for disinfection), extended wear (can be worn nonstop for up to thirty days), and disposable (replaced every day or every two weeks).

STEROID Any of numerous naturally occurring or synthetic, fat-soluble organic compounds, including sterols, bile acids, sex hormones, adrenocortical hormones, and the precursors of certain vitamins. Used in dry eye therapy as topical drops to reduce and eliminate inflammation.

STEVENS-JOHNSON SYNDROME A severe inflammatory eruption of the skin and mucous membranes, rather like a very serious burn; often occurs in children and young adults following an infection or as a reaction to drugs.

STRABISMUS A problem caused by one or more improperly functioning eye muscles resulting in misalignment of the eyes.

STROMA The layer of cornea under the epithelium that accounts for 90 percent of the corneal thickness and is optically clear under normal conditions to allow the passage of light to reach the retina.

STY A small tender bump in the eyelid caused by obstruction of an oil-producing or meibomian gland.

SUBCONJUNCTIVAL HEMORRHAGE Bleeding when a small blood vessel within the conjunctiva breaks.

SUPERIOR LIMBIC KERATOCONJUNCTIVITIS Inflammation of the superior (top) part of the eye including the conjunctiva and upper part of the cornea; can occur in dry eye or in association with thyroid conditions.

SURGICENTER An outpatient surgical facility.

SYNDROME A group of signs and symptoms that often occur simultaneously and characterize an abnormality.

TARSORRHAPHY An operation to reduce the size of the opening between the eyelids by stitching the outer eyelids together.

TBUT (TEAR BREAK-UP TIME) TEST A means of evaluating the time it takes for the tear film to destabilize on the surface of the eye.

TEAR CLEARANCE (also **tear turnover**) The rate at which tears are cleared from the surface of the eye.

TEAR CLEARANCE TEST A way of judging how effectively the eye removes old tears and is replenished with new tears; it can indicate abnormal aqueous tear production.

TEAR FILM The liquid that resides or flows over the surface of the eye; three layers as follows: outer oily layer, mostly produced by the meibomian glands (lipid layer); a salt-watery middle layer, mostly produced by the lacrimal glands (watery layer); and an inner mucus layer secreted by goblet cells in the conjunctiva (mucin layer).

TEAR GLAND One of the glands (lacrimal, meibomian) that produce the water, lipids, and other materials that constitute the tear film.

THERMOCAUTERY OF PUNCTA The use of heat to burn puncta to achieve a narrowing or closure of the punctal opening.

THYGESON'S KERATITIS A disorder of the cornea that causes irritation and fluctuating vision and may be confused with dry eye.

TOPIC SOFT CONTACT LENS A soft lens designed to correct astigmatism as well as nearsightedness or farsightedness.

TOXICITY The condition of being poisonous or injurious; also the degree to which a substance is toxic.
TRANSILLUMINATOR A device used to view the meibomian glands within the eyelids.
TREPHINE An instrument used to perform LASEK surgery.
TRICHIASIS A disease in which the eyelashes become misdirected, growing inward toward the surface of the eye instead of outward, and thus irritate or abrade the ocular surface. Can cause discomfort and possibly corneal ulceration and perforation.

VASOCONSTRICTOR A drug that constricts blood vessels in the eyes, thus eliminating redness.
VERNAL KERATOCONJUNCTIVITIS A rare ocular allergic disorder that mostly affects boys under age 10; most often seen in hot or polluted climates.
VITREOUS CHAMBER The large, round area behind the lens, which forms the "ball" of the eyeball; filled with vitreous humor.
VITREOUS HUMOR A gelatinous liquid located in the vitreous chamber.

WATERY TEAR One of the tears secreted by the lacrimal glands; they compose the middle (thickest) layer of the tear film.

XEROPHTHALMIA Dry eye caused by vitamin-A deficiency. The conjunctiva and cornea become nonwettable, which if not corrected can lead to corneal ulceration, perforation, and blindness.

# RESOURCES

## GENERAL HEALTH REFERENCE BOOKS

It is worthwhile to have one or two respected health guides on your home bookshelf to reference family health and medical issues, including problems relating to the eye. Here are a few excellent general resources.

Beers, Mark H., et al. (eds.), *The Merck Manual of Medical Information*. New York: Pocket Books, 2003.

Clayman, Charles B., *The American Medical Association Encyclopedia of Medicine*. New York: Random House, 1989.

Editors of the Johns Hopkins Health after 50 Newsletter, *The Johns Hopkins Medical Handbook: The 100 Major Medical Disorders of People over the Age of 50*. New York: Rebus (distributed by Random House), 1992.

Editors of the University of California at Berkeley Wellness Letter, *The New Wellness Encyclopedia*. Boston: Houghton Mifflin, 1995.

Kirchheimer, Sid, and editors of *Prevention Magazine* health books. *The Doctors Book of Home Remedies II*. Emmaus, Pennsylvania: Rodale Press, 1993.

Leikin, Jerrold B., and Martin S. Lipsky, *The American Medical Association Complete Medical Encyclopedia*. New York: Random House, 2003.

Mayo Clinic staff, *The Mayo Clinic Family Health Book*. New York: HarperCollins, 2003.

BOOKS ON DRY EYE SYNDROME AND RELATED TOPICS

These are the books that I used to prepare *Reversing Dry Eye Syndrome*. Some are intended for ophthalmologists and other eye care professionals and thus are very technical, and some are very expensive. You may be able to find them in your local library and reference them for your specific problems regarding dry eye.

Berube, Margery S., and eds., *The American Heritage Stedman's Medical Dictionary*. Boston: Houghton Mifflin, 2002.

Frey, William, *Crying: The Mystery of Tears*. Minneapolis: Winston Press, 1985.

Holland, Edward J., and Mark J. Mannis (eds.), *Ocular Surface Disease: Medical and Surgical Management*. New York: Springer-Verlag, 2002.

Hoang-Xuan, Thanh, Christophe Baudouin, and Catherine Creuzot-Garcher, *Inflammatory Diseases of the Conjunctiva*. New York: Thieme, 2001.

Li, Alain Wan Po, et al., *OTC Medications: Symptoms and Treatments of Common Illnesses*. Blackwell Science, 1997.

Parker, James N., and Philip M. Parker (eds.), *The 2002 Official Patient's Sourcebook on Dry Eye: A Revised and Updated Directory for the Internet Age*. San Diego: ICON Health Publications, 2002.

Pflugfelder, Stephen C., Roger W. Beuerman, and Michael E. Stern (eds.), *Dry Eye and Ocular Surface Disorders*. New York: Marcel Dekker, 2004.

## GENERAL HEALTH NEWSLETTERS

Several fine health newsletters are readily available. Here are three to consider.

*Bottom Line's Daily Health News*
This daily health newsletter is published online by BottomLine-Secrets and Boardroom, Inc.; it is sent free via email. A lively newsletter that reports on trends in health for all ages. To order, contact *www.bottomlinesecrets.com/cust.service/contact,* or Boardroom, Inc., 281 Tresser Boulevard, Stamford, Connecticut 06901-3246; Attn: Web Team.

*Johns Hopkins Health after 50 Newsletter*
This newsletter, from one of America's most prestigious health centers, focuses on health issues of concern to people over age 50. Edited by experts from a wide range of fields, this monthly eight-page publication offers commentary on the latest developments in modern health care. Potentially of special interest to dry eye sufferers, since the majority are over age 50. To subscribe, visit *http://www.hopkinsafter50.com/html/contact/cuHome.php*.

*University of California at Berkeley Wellness Letter*
One of America's most authoritative health newsletters, this publication incorporates expertise not only from the School of Public Health at the University of California, but from researchers, doctors, and wellness experts from around the world. It provides up-to-date news stories, health trends, hints and tips, and other information on all aspects of health for all ages. The eight-page newsletter is published monthly and is not expensive. A lively and responsible general health overview. To subscribe, visit *http://www.wellnessletter.com*.

## HELPFUL WEBSITES

Many useful websites with information about dry eye syndrome can be found online. Many of them are valuable, particularly those associated with important medical institutions such as the Johns Hopkins Hospital and the Mayo Clinic. (To get to these websites, use an efficient search engine such as Google; you'll find them very quickly.) Although it is important to read as much as you can about dry eye, always consult with your eye doctor before using any medication or procedure recommended online.

Below are two websites that you may find helpful.

### The Schepens Eye Research Institute

*www.theschepens.org*
The Schepens Eye Research Institute at Harvard University, Cambridge, Massachusetts, is the largest independent eye research institute in America. It has contributed greatly to knowledge of the human body in general, and to ophthalmology in particular. The website offers fact sheets on various diseases and disorders, including dry eye.

### The Boston Scleral Lens

*www.bostonsight.org/aboutlens.htm*
A site that provides complete information on the Boston scleral lens.

## ARTICLES IN JOURNALS AND BOOKS

The following is a list of documents used to prepare the various chapters of this book. Again, most of these references are intended for ophthalmologists and other eye care medical professionals. However, since information for the general reader is so scarce at the moment, I include the citations here. You can find many of these journals in a large urban or university library, and in some cases online.

## Chapter 1. What Is Dry Eye Syndrome, and Who Gets It?

Abelson, Mark B., and Jason Casavant, "Give Dry Eye a One-Two Punch," *Review of Ophthalmology,* March 2003, 74–77.

Bjerrum, K. B., "Keratoconjunctivitis Sicca and Primary Sjögren's Syndrome in a Danish Population aged 30–60 Years," *Acta Ophthalmologica Scandinavica* 1997, vol. 75, 281–286.

Charles, Lynda, "Dry Eye Syndrome Can Severely Affect Quality of Life," Special Section: Dry Eye, *Ophthalmology Times,* May 15, 2005, 17.

Lemp, Michael, A., "Dry Eye, Climate and Seasons," *Refractive Eyecare for Ophthalmologists,* November 2003, 24.

McCarty, C. A., et al., "The Epidemiology of Dry Eye in Melbourne, Australia," *Ophthalmology,* June 1998, 1114–19.

Pflugfelder, Stephen C., "Anti-inflammatory Therapy of Dry Eye," *The Ocular Surface,* January 2003, 31–36.

——. Preface and Chapter 1 in Pflugfelder, Beuerman, and Stern (eds.), *Dry Eye and Ocular Surface Disorders*. New York: Marcel Dekker, 2004.

Salinger, Clifford, "Dry Eye: It's a Brand New Day," *Ophthalmology Management,* November 2003, 101–108.

Shimmura, S., Shimazaki, J., and Tsubota, K., "Results of a Population Based Questionnaire on the Symptoms and Lifestyles Associated with Dry Eye," *Cornea,* July 1999, 408–411.

## Chapter 2. An Overview of the Eye

Beers, Mark H., et al. (eds.), *The Merck Manual of Medical Information*. New York: Pocket Books, 2003, passim.

Clayman, Charles B., *The American Medical Association Encyclopedia of Medicine*. New York: Random House, 1989, passim.

Editors of the Johns Hopkins Health after 50 Newsletter, "The Eyes," in *The Johns Hopkins Medical Handbook: The 100 Major Medical Disorders of People over the Age of 50*. New York: Rebus (distributed by Random House), 1992, 259–275.

Editors of the University of California at Berkeley Wellness Letter, "Eye Care," in *The New Wellness Encyclopedia*. Boston: Houghton Mifflin, 1995, 327–339.

Kirchheimer, Sid, and editors of *Prevention Magazine* health books. "Dry Eyes," in *The Doctors Book of Home Remedies II*. Emmaus, Pennsylvania: Rodale Press, 1993, 171–174.

Larson, David D., and eds., "The Eyes," in *The Mayo Clinic Family Health Book*. New York: William Morrow, 1989, 731–781.

### Chapter 3. The Dry Eye

Abelson, M. B., Jason Casavant, and Lauren Nalfy, "The Secret(agogue) Is Out," *Review of Ophthalmology,* November 2002, 72–76.

Abelson, M. B., Kate Humphrey, and Darlene A. Dartt, "Mucin: What You Don't Know May Help You," *Review of Ophthalmology,* January 2003, 70–73.

Beuerman, Roger W., et al., "The Lacrimal Functional Unit," in Pflugfelder, Beuerman, and Stern (eds.), *Dry Eye and Ocular Surface Disorders*. New York: Marcel Dekker, 2004, 11–39.

Bron, A. J., and J. M. Tiffany, "The Contribution of Meibomian Disease to Dry Eye," *The Ocular Surface,* April 2004, 149–164.

Dartt, Darlene A., "Dysfunctional Neural Regulation of Lacrimal Gland Secretion and Its Role in the Pathogenesis of Dry Eye Syndrome," *The Ocular Surface,* April 2004, 76–79.

Frey, William, *Crying: The Mystery of Tears*. Minneapolis: Winston Press, 1985.

Levoy, Gregg, "Tears that Speak," *Psychology Today,* July–August 1988, 8, 10.

McCulley, James P., and Ward E. Shine, "Meibomian Gland Function and the Tear Lipid Layer," *The Ocular Surface,* July 2003, 97–106.

Murube, Juan, "Crocodile Tears," *The Ocular Surface,* April 2005, 69–71.

Nakamori, Katsu, et al., "Blinking Is Controlled Primarily by Ocular Surface Conditions," *American Journal of Ophthalmology,* July 1997, 24–30.

Nicolaides, N., et al., "Meibomian Gland Studies: Comparison of Steer and Human Lipids," *Investigative Ophthalmology and Visual Science,* 1981, vol. 20, 522–536.

Stern, Michael E., Roger W. Beuerman, and Stephen C. Pflugfelder, "The Normal Tear Film and Ocular Surface," in Pflugfelder, Beuerman, and Stern (eds.), *Dry Eye and Ocular Surface Disorders.* New York: Marcel Dekker, 2004, 40–61.

Stern, Michael E., et al., "The Pathology of Dry Eye: The Interaction Between the Ocular Surface and the Lacrimal Glands," *Cornea,* 1998, 584–589.

Tomlinson, Alan, and Santosh Khanal, "Assessment of Tear Film Dynamics, Quantification Approach," *The Ocular Surface,* April 2005, 81–95.

Tsubota, Kazuo, Scheffer C. G. Tseng, and Michael L. Nordlund, "Anatomy and Physiology of the Ocular Surface," in Holland and Mannis (eds.), *Ocular Surface Disease: Medical and Surgical Management.* New York: Springer-Verlag, 2002, 3–27.

## Chapter 4. The Causes

Blehm, Clayton, et al., "Computer Vision Syndrome: A Review," *Survey of Ophthalmology,* May–June 2005, 253–262.

Duenwald, Mary, "For Dry Eye Sufferers, Lots of Tears Bring Major Relief," *New York Times,* September 13, 2005.

Editors of the University of California at Berkeley Wellness Letter, "Dry Eyes That Cry," September 2005.

Foulks, Gary N., "Blepharitis: Lid Margin Disease and the Ocular Surface," in Holland and Mannis (eds.), *Ocular Surface Disease: Medical and Surgical Management.* New York: Springer-Verlag, 2002, 39–48.

Gilbard, Jeffrey P., "Dry Eye: Natural History, Diagnosis, and Treatment," *Ophthalmology Management,* November 2003, S1–S6.

Groves, Nancy, "Dry Eye Linked to Diabetes: Decreased Corneal Sensation," *Ophthalmology Times,* May 15, 2005, 34.

Kaiserman, Igor, et al., "Dry Eye in Diabetic Patients," *American Journal of Ophthalmology,* March 2005, 498–503.

Kim, Terry, and B. Alyse Khosla-Gupta, "Chemical and Thermal Injuries to the Ocular Surface," in Holland and Mannis (eds.), *Ocular Surface Disease: Medical and Surgical Management.* New York: Springer-Verlag, 2002, 100–112.

Kruse, Frederick E., "Classification of Ocular Surface Disease," in Edward J. Holland and Mark J. Mannis (eds.), *Ocular Surface Disease: Medical and Surgical Management.* New York: Spring-Verlag, 2002, 16–36.

Pflugfelder, Stephen C., and Abraham Solomon, "Dry Eye," in Holland and Mannis (eds.), *Ocular Surface Disease: Medical and Surgical Management.* New York: Springer Verlag, 2002, 49–57.

Pflugfelder, Stephen C., et al., "RRS Ocular Surface Roundtable," *Review of Refractive Surgery,* August 2003, 19–25.

Spencer, J., "The Blackberry Squint: Growing PDA Use Hurts Eyes," *Wall Street Journal,* April 25, 2006.

Tauber, Joseph, "Autoimmune Diseases Affecting the Ocular Surface," in Holland and Mannis (eds.), *Ocular Surface Disease: Medical and Surgical Management.* New York: Springer-Verlag, 2002, 113–127.

Tsubota, Kazuo, Scheffer C. G. Tseng, and Michael L. Nordlund, "Anatomy and Physiology of the Ocular Surface," in Holland and Mannis (eds.), *Ocular Surface Disease: Medical and Surgical Management.* New York: Springer-Verlag, 2002, 3–27.

## Chapter 5. Aging and Gender

Cermak, Jennifer M., et al., "Is Complete Androgen Insensitivity Syndrome Associated with Alterations in the Meibomian Gland and Ocular Surface?" *Cornea,* 2003, vol. 22, no. 6, 516–521.

Coleman, Anne L., et al., "Higher Risk of Multiple Falls Among Elderly Women Who Lose Visual Acuity," *Ophthalmology,* May 2004, 857–862.

Goto, Eiki, et al., "Impaired Functional Visual Acuity of Dry Eye Patients," *American Journal of Ophthalmology,* February 2002, 181–186.

Krenzer, Kathleen L., et al., "Effect of Androgen Deficiency on the Human Meibomian Gland and Ocular Surface," *Journal of Clinical Endocrinology and Metabolism,* 2002, vol. 85, no. 12, 4874–82.

Mathers, William D., et al., "Menopause and Tear Function: The Influence of Prolactin and Sex Hormones on Human Tear Production," *Cornea,* 1998, vol. 17, no. 4, 353–358.

Mircheff, Austin, K., "Understanding the Causes of Lacrimal Insufficiency: Implications for Treatment and Prevention of Dry Eye Syndrome," Paper for Research to Prevent Blindness Science Writers Seminar, 1993.

Moss, Scott E., Ronald Klein, and Barbara E. K. Klein, "Incidence of Dry Eye in an Older Population," *Archives of Ophthalmology,* March 2004, 369–373.

Obata, Hrioto, et al., "Histopathologic Study of the Human Lacrimal Gland: Statistical Analysis with Special Reference to Aging," *Ophthalmology,* April 1995, 678–686.

Pflugfelder, Stephen C., "Hormonal Deficiencies and Dry Eye," *Archives of Ophthalmology,* February 2004, 273–274.

Pflugfelder, Stephen C., and Abraham Solomon, "Dry Eye," in Holland and Mannis (eds.), *Ocular Surface Disease: Medical and Surgical Management.* New York: Springer-Verlag, 2002, 49–57.

Sato, Elcio H., and David A. Sullivan, "Comparative Influence of Steroid Hormones and Immunosuppressive Agents on Autoimmune Expression in Lacrimal Glands of a Female Mouse Model of Sjögren's Syndrome," *Investigative Ophthalmology and Visual Science,* April 1994, 2632–42.

Schaumberg, Debra A., et al., "Hormone Replacement Therapy and Dry Eye Syndrome," *Journal of American Medical Association,* November 7, 2001, 2114–19.

——. "Prevalence of Dry Eye Syndrome Among U.S. Women," *American Journal of Ophthalmology,* 2003, vol. 136, no. 2, 318–326.

Schein, Oliver D., et al., "Prevalence of Dry Eye Among the Elderly," *American Journal of Ophthalmology,* 1997, vol. 124, no. 6, 723–728.

Scott, Garrett, et al., "Combined Esterified Estrogen and Methyltestosterone Treatment for Dry Eye Syndrome in Postmenopausal Women," *American Journal of Ophthalmology,* 2005, vol. 139, 1109–10.

Sloan, Frank A., et al., "Effects of Changes in Self-Reported Vision on Cognitive, Affective, and Functional Status and Living Arrangements Among the Elderly," *American Journal of Ophthalmology,* October 2005, 618–627.

Smith, Janine A., et al., "Dry Eye Signs and Symptoms in Women with Premature Ovarian Failure," *Archives of Ophthalmology,* February 2004, 151–156.

Sullivan, Benjamin D., et al., "Complete Androgen Insensitivity Syndrome: Effect on Human Meibomian Gland Secretions," *Archives of Ophthalmology,* December 2002, 1689–99.

Sullivan, David A., "Sex and Sex Steroid Influences on Dry Eye Syndrome," in Pflugfelder, Beuerman, and Stern (eds.), *Dry Eye and Ocular Surface Disorders.* New York: Marcel Dekker, 2004, 165–190.

——. "Tearful Relationships? Sex, Hormones, the Lacrimal Gland, and Aqueous-Deficient Dry Eye," *The Ocular Surface,* April 2004, 92–123.

Tamer, Cengaver, et al., "Tear Film Tests in Parkinson's Disease Patients," *Ophthalmology,* October 2005, 1795–1800.

## Chapter 6. Allergies, Toxicities, and Other Sensitivities

Abelson, Mark B., and Kate Fink, "What Makes a Patient Allergic?" *Review of Ophthalmology,* March 2005, 74–76.

Abelson, Mark B., Lisa Smith, and Matthew Chapin, "Ocular Allergic Disease: Mechanisms, Disease Sub-types, Treatment," *The Ocular Surface,* July 2003, 127–149.

——. *The Allergy Report.* Website of the American Academy of Allergy, Ashthma, and Immunology, 1996–2005.

Arbes, S. J., et al., "Dog Allergen and Cat Allergen in U.S. Homes: Results from the National Survey of Lead and Allergens in Housing," *Journal of Allergy and Clinical Immunology,* July 2004, 111–117.

Basu, P. K., et al., "The Effect of Cigarette Smoke on the Human Tear Film," *Canadian Journal of Ophthalmology,* 1978, vol. 13., no. 22, 22–26.

Baudouin, C. "Focus 8. Role of Inflammation in Dry Eye Syndrome," in Thanh Hoang-Xuan, Christophe Baudouin, and Catherine Creuzot-Garcher, *Inflammatory Diseases of the Conjunctiva.* New York: Thieme, 2001, 157–160.

——. "Iatrogenic Disorders of the Ocular Surface," in Hoang-Xuan, Baudouin, and Creuzot-Garcher, *Inflammatory Diseases of the Conjunctiva.* New York: Thieme, 2001, 133–142.

Berkow, Robert, et al., "Allergic Reactions," *The Merck Manual of Medical Information.* Whitehouse Station, New Jersey: Merck & Company, 1997, 962–971.

Daly, Rich, and others, "More Effective Treatments Better Control Allergies"; "To Combat Allergies in Children, It's Avoidance, Then Treatment"; "Responding to Non-Prescription Allergy Medication Complications"; "Attacking Allergens a Must for Allergic Contact Lens Wearers"; and "Best Strategies to Treat CL Users That Have Allergies," *EyeWorld,* February 2005, 36–48.

Gonzalez, Jeanne Michelle, "Distinguishing Dry Eye from Ocular Allergy: Careful History Should Tell the Story," *Ocular Surgery News,* February 15, 2004, 38.

Goto, Eiki, et al., "Impaired Functional Visual Acuity of Dry Eye Patients," *American Journal of Ophthalmology,* February 2002, 181–186.

Hannouche, D., and T. Hoang-Xuan, "Allergic Conjunctivitis," in Hoang-Xuan, Baudouin, and Creuzot-Garcher, *Inflammatory Diseases of the Conjunctiva.* New York: Thieme, 2001, 51–70.

Hoang-Xuan, T., "Ocular Rosacea," in Hoang-Xuan, Baudouin, and Creuzot-Garcher, *Inflammatory Diseases of the Conjunctiva.* New York: Thieme, 2001, 97–108.

Ishida, Reiko, et al., "The Application of a New Continuous Functional Visual Acuity Measurement System in Dry Eye Syndromes," *American Journal of Ophthalmology,* February 2005, 253–258.

Lanier, Bob O. "Understanding Allergic Reaction," *Review of Ophthalmology,* April 2005, 82B–82H.

Nakamori, Katsu, et al., "Blinking Is Controlled Primarily by Ocular Surface Conditions," *American Journal of Ophthalmology,* July 1997, 24–30.

Pflugfelder, Stephen C., et al., "RRS Ocular Surface Roundtable: Treating Allergy," *Review of Refractive Surgery,* August 2003, 24–25.

Raizman, Michael B., "Topical Therapy for Ocular Allergy: Making Sense of the Available Drugs," *Therapeutic Updates in Ophthalmology,* 2005, vol. 6, no. 3, 3, 8.

——. "Dry Eye Fact Sheet." Website of The Schepens Eye Research Institute, Harvard University, Cambridge, Massachusetts, *www.theschepens.org.*

## Chapter 7. Contact Lenses

American Academy of Ophthalmology Refractive Errors Panel (Sid Mandelbaum et al.), "Refractive Errors," 2002, 7–8, 36–38.

Gilbard, Jeffrey P., Kathleen L. Gray, and Scott R. Rossi, "A Proposed Mechanism for Increased Tear-Film Osmolarity in Contact Lens Wearers," *American Journal of Ophthalmology,* October 1986, 505–507.

## Chapter 8. LASIK and Other Refractive Surgeries

Abelson, Mark B., Lisa Smith, and Kate King, "The Best Corneal Surface for LASIK," *Review of Ophthalmology,* January 2004, 68–70.

American Academy of Ophthalmology Refractive Errors Panel (Sid Mandelbaum et al.), "Refractive Errors," 2002, 10–31.

Beers, Mark H., et al. (eds.), "Refractive Disorders," *The Merck Manual of Medical Information*. New York: Pocket Books, 2003, 1161–64.

Calvillo, Martha P., et al., "Cornea Reinnervation after LASIK: Prospective 3-Year Longitudinal Study," *Investigative Ophthalmology and Visual Science,* November 2004, 3991–96.

Donnenfeld, Eric, "Minimizing Post-LASIK Dry Eye," *Ophthalmology Management,* September 2004, 57–59, 61, 63–64.

Donnenfeld, E., et al., "The Effect of Hinge Position on Cornea Sensation and Dry Eye after LASIK," *Ophthalmology,* 2003, vol. 110, 1023–30.

*Eye World* staff and Scheffer C. G. Tseng, "Dry Eye: A Link With LASIK?" *EyeWorld,* September 2005.

Huang, Bo, et al., "The Effect of Punctal Occlusion on Wavefront Aberrations in Dry Eye Patients after Laser in Situ Keratomileusis," *American Journal of Ophthalmology,* January 2004, 52–61.

Nejima, Ryohei, et al., "Corneal Barrier Function, Tear Film Stability, and Corneal Sensation after PRK and LASIK," *American Journal of Ophthalmology,* January 2005, 64–71.

Pallikaris, Ioannis, et al., "Epi-LASIK: Preliminary Clinical Results of an Alternative Surface Ablation Procedure," *Journal of Cataract and Refractive Surgery,* May 2005, 879–885.

Pflugfelder, Stephen C., et al., "RRS Ocular Surface Roundtable," *Review of Refractive Surgery,* August 2003, 19–25.

Sabbagh, Leslie B., "Optimizing the Ocular Surface: Translating Theory into Refractive Practice," *Review of Refractive Surgery,* August 2004, 9–20.

Solomon, Renee, Eric D. Donnenfeld, and Henry D. Perry, "The Effects of LASIK on the Ocular Surface," *The Ocular Surface,* January 2004, 34–44.

Taneri, Suphi, James Zieske, and Dimitri Azar, "Evolution Techniques, Clinical Outcomes, and Pathophysiology of LASEK: Review of the Literature," *Survey of Ophthalmology,* November–December 2004, 576–602.

Toda, Ikuko, et al., "Ocular Surface Treatment Before Laser in situ Keratomileusis (LASIK) in Patients with Severe Dry Eye," *Journal of Refractive Surgery,* May-June 2004, 270–275.

Wilson, Steven E., and faculty/editorial board, Postgraduate Institute for Medicine, "LASIK and Dry Eyes: LASIK-Induced Neurotrophic Epitheliopathy," *Review of Refractive Surgery,* September 2000, 49–56.

Yamane, Nayori, et al., "Ocular Higher-Order Aberrations and Contrast Sensitivity after Conventional LASIK," *Investigative Ophthalmology and Visual Science,* November 2004, 3986–90.

Yu, Edward Y. W., et al., "Effect of Laser in situ Keratomileusis on Tear Stability," *Ophthalmology,* December 2000, 2131–35.

## Chapter 9. The Diagnosis

Afonso, Adolfo A., et al., "Correlation of Tear Fluorescein Clearance and Schirmer Test Scores with Ocular Irritation Symptoms," *Ophthalmology,* April 1999, 803–810.

Chalmers, Robin L., et al., "The Agreement Between Self-Assessment and Clinician Assessment of Dry Eye Severity," *Cornea,* October 2005, 804–810.

De Paiva, Cintia S., and Stephen C. Pflugfelder, "Diagnostic Approaches to Lacrimal Keratoconjunctivitis," in Pflugfelder, Beuerman, and Stern (eds.), *Dry Eye and Ocular Surface Disorders.* New York: Marcel Dekker, 2004, 269–308.

Dogru, Murat, and Kazuo Tsubota, "New Insights into the Diagnosis and Treatment of Dry Eye," *The Ocular Surface,* April 2004, 59–75.

Gilbard, Jeffrey P., "Dry Eye: Natural History, Diagnosis, and Treatment," *Ophthalmology Management,* November 2003, S1–S8.

Miljanovic, Biljana, et al., "Relation Between Dietary n-3 and n-6 Fatty Acids and Clinically Diagnosed Dry Eye Syndrome in Women," *American Journal of Clinical Nutrition,* October 2005, 887–893.

Nichols, Kelly K., Jason J. Nichols, and G. Lynn Mitchell, "The Lack of Association Between Signs and Symptoms in Patients with Dry Eye Disease," *Cornea,* November 2004, 762–770.

Pflugfelder, Stephen C., et al., "Evaluation of Subjective Assessments and Objective Diagnostic Tests for Diagnosing Tear-Film Disorders Known to Cause Ocular Irritation," *Cornea,* January 1998, 38–56.

Schiffman, Rhett M., et al., "Reliability and Validity of the Ocular Surface Disease Index," *Archives of Ophthalmology,* May 2000, 615–621.

——. "Utility Assessment Among Patients with Dry Eye Disease," *Ophthalmology,* July 2003, 1412–19.

## Chapter 10. Treatment

Abelson, Mark B., and Jason Casvant, "Give Dry Eye a One-Two Punch," *Review of Ophthalmology,* March 2003, 74–77.

Abelson, Mark B., and Anne Giovanni, "How to Specify Artificial Tears," *Review of Ophthalmology,* July 1997, 108–109.

Abelson, Mark B., and Susan Washburn, "The Downside of Tear Preservatives," *Review of Ophthalmology,* May 2001, 102–106.

Abelson, Mark B., Jason Casvant, and Lauren Nalfy, "The Secret(agogue) Is Out," *Review of Ophthalmology,* November 2002, 72–76.

Abelson, Mark B., et al., "Dry Eye: How to Ask the Right Questions," *Review of Ophthalmology,* October 2005, 126–128.

Barber, Laurie D., et al., "Phase III: Safety Evaluation of Cyclosporine 0.1% Ophthalmic Emulsion Administered Twice Daily to Dry Eye Disease Patients for up to 3 Years," *Ophthalmology,* October 2005, 1790–94.

Baxter, Stephanie A., and M. D. Laibson, "Punctal Plugs in the Management of Dry Eyes," *The Ocular Surface,* October 2004, 255–265.

Dhaliwal, Deepinder K., and others, *An Algorithm-Based Approach to the Diagnosis and Treatment of Dry Eye,* Supplement to Refractive Eyecare, October 2005, 1–19.

Di Pascuale, M. D., et al., "Clinical Characteristics of Conjunctivochalasis with or without Aqueous Tear Deficiency," *British Journal of Ophthalmology,* vol. 88, 2004, 388–392.

Dogru, Murat, and Kazuo Tsubota, "New Insights into the Diagnosis and Treatment of Dry Eye," *The Ocular Surface,* April 2004, 59–75.

Donnenfeld, Eric, "The Role of Nutrition in the Management of Dry Eye," *Refractive Eyecare for Ophthalmologists,* June 2003, 23–25.

Erasmus, Udo, *Fats That Heal, Fats That Kill.* Burnaby, British Columbia, Canada: Alive Books, 1993.

Georgiadis, Nick S., and Chryssa D. Terzidou, "Epiphora Caused by Conjunctivochalasis," *Cornea,* August 2001, 619–621.

Groves, Nancy, "Nutritional Supplement Stimulates Aqueous Tear Production," *Ophthalmology Times,* May 15, 2003.

Hardten, David R., Robert J. Noecker, and Stephen C. Pflugfelder, "The Current Consensus in the Management of Chronic Dry Eye," *Ophthalmology Times,* July 15, 2005, suppl. 11, 1–8.

Kim, Bryan M., Smajo S. Osmanovic, and Deepak P. Edward, "Pygenic Granulomas after Silcone Punctal Plugs: A Clinical and Histopathologic Study," *American Journal of Ophthalmology,* April 2005, 678–684.

Kojima, Takashi, et al., "The Effect of Autologous Serum Eyedrops in the Treatment of Severe Dry Eye Disease: A Prospective Randomized Case-Control Study," *American Journal of Ophthalmology,* February 2005, 242–246.

Kronemyer, Bob, "Dry Eye Successfully Treated with Oral Flaxseed Oil," *Ocular Surgery News,* October 15, 2000, 147.

Lee, Judith, "Better-Looking Goggles Might Work Better, Too," *Review of Ophthalmology,* June 2005, 100–101.

Lemp, Michael A., "Mucin Secretagogues in Dry Eye," *Refractive Eyecare for Ophthalmologists,* June 2003, 26.

——. "New Strategies in the Treatment of Dry-Eye States," *Cornea,* November 1999, 625–632.

Marsh, Peter, and Stephen C. Pflugfelder, "Topical Nonpreserved Methylprednisolone Therapy for Keratoconjunctivitis Sicca in Sjögren's Syndrome," *Ophthalmology,* April 1999, 811–816.

McDonnell, P. J., et al., "The Dysfunctional Tear Syndrome Group" (a modified Delphi technique to obtain consensus on the treatment of dysfunctional tear syndrome). Poster presented at the annual meeting of the Association for Research in Vision and Ophthalmology, April 25–29, 2004, Fort Lauderdale, Florida.

Meadows, David, et al., "Science Behind Today's Artificial Tears," *Ophthalmology Management,* June 2005, 29–30.

Meller, Daniel, and Scheffer C. G. Tseng, "Conjunctivochalasis: Literature Review and Possible Pathophysiology," *Survey of Ophthalmology,* November-December 1998, 225–232.

Meller, Daniel, et al., "Amniotic Membrane Transplantation for Symptomatic Conjunctivochalasis Refractory to Medical Treatments," *Cornea,* November 2002, 796–803.

Miljanovic, Biljana, et al., "Relation Between Dietary n-3 and n-6 Fatty Acids and Clinically Diagnosed Dry Eye Syndrome in Women," *American Journal of Clinical Nutrition,* October 2005, 887–893.

Montes-Mico, Robert, Araceli Caliz, and Jorge L. Alio, "Changes in Ocular Aberrations after Instillation of Artificial Tears in Dry-Eye Patients," *Journal of Cataract and Refractive Surgery,* August 2004, 1649–52.

Moss, Scot E., Ronald Klein, and Barbara E. K. Klein, "Prevalence of and Risk Factors for Dry Eye Syndrome," *Archives of Ophthalmology,* September 2000, 1264–68.

Murube, Juan, "Characteristics and Etiology of Conjunctivochalasis: Historical Perspective," *The Ocular Surface,* January 2005, 7–12.

Nichols, Kelly K., Jason J. Nichols, and G. Lynn Mitchell, "The Lack of Association Between Signs and Symptoms in Patients with Dry Eye Disease," *Cornea,* November 2004, 762–770.

O'Brien, Terrence P., "Flaxseed Oil: The Not-So-Hidden Secret," *Cataract and Refractive Surgery Today,* February 2003, 61–62.

Pflugfelder, Stephen C., "Anti-inflammatory Therapy of Dry Eye," *The Ocular Surface,* January 2003, 31–36.

Pflugfelder, Stephen C., and Michael E. Stern, "Therapy of Lacrimal Keratoconjunctivitis," in Pflugfelder, Beuerman, and Stern (eds.), *Dry Eye and Ocular Surface Disorders.* New York: Marcel Dekker, 2004, 309–324.

Pflugfelder, Stephen, et al., "A Randomized, Double-Masked Placebo-Controlled, Multicenter Comparison of Loteprednol Etabonate Ophthalmic Suspension, 0.5%, and Placebo for Treatment of Keratoconjunctivitis Sicca in Patients with Delayed Tear Clearance," *American Journal of Ophthalmology,* September 2004, 444–457.

Pflugfelder, Stephen C., et al., "Evaluation of Subjective Assessments and Objective Diagnostic Tests for Diagnosing Tear-Film Disorders Known to Cause Ocular Irritation," *Cornea,* January 1998, 38–51.

Salinger, Clifford, "Dry Eye: It's a Brand New Day," *Ophthalmology Management,* November 2003, 101–108.

Tananuvat, Napaporn, et al., "Controlled Study of the Use of Autologous Serum in Dry Eye Patients," November 2001, *Cornea,* 802–806.

Yen, Michael T., "Surgical Therapy for Ocular Surface Disorders," in Pflugfelder, Beuerman, and Stern (eds.), *Dry Eye and Ocular Surface Disorders.* New York: Marcel Dekker, 2004, 325–342.

### Chapter 11. Remedies for Home and Work

Abelson, Mark B., G. Ousler, and A. Plumer, "Heighten Dry-Eye Situational Awareness," *Review of Ophthalmology,* December 2005, 64–66.

Basu, P. K., et al., "The Effect of Cigarette Smoke on the Human Tear Film," *Canadian Journal of Ophthalmology,* January 1978, 22–26.

Blehm, Clayton, et al., "Computer Vision Syndrome: A Review," *Survey of Ophthalmology,* May-June 2005, 253–262.

Donnenfeld, Eric, "The Role of Nutrition in the Management of Dry Eye," *Refractive Eyecare for Ophthalmologists,* June 2003, 23–25.

Groves, Nancy, "Nutritional Supplement Stimulates Aqueous Tear Production," *Ophthalmology Times,* May 15, 2003.

Kirchheimer, Sid, and the editors of *Prevention Magazine* health books, "Dry Eyes," in *The Doctors Book of Home Remedies II.* Emmaus, Pennsylvania: Rodale Press, 1993, 171–174.

Lemp, Michael A., "Dry Eye, Climate and Seasons," *Refractive Eyecare for Ophthalmologists,* November 2003, 24.

Lipner, Maxine, "Consider These Factors Addressing Dry Eye in Menopausal Women," *EyeWorld,* May 2005, 43–44.

Salinger, Clifford, "Dry Eye: It's a Brand New Day," *Ophthalmology Management,* November 2003, 101–108.

# INDEX